OPHTHALMIC NURSING

OPHTHALMIC NURSING

A.K. Khurana
M.S., C.T.O. (London)
Associate Professor,
Department of Ophthalmology,
Postgraduate Institute of Medical Sciences,
Rohtak - 124001 (Haryana)

Foreword by
Shashi Sood
M.Sc. (Nursing)
Principal, School of Nursing,
PGIMS, Rohtak

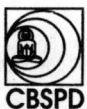

CBSPD

CBS Publishers & Distributors Pvt Ltd

New Delhi • Bengaluru • Chennai • Kochi • Kolkata • Lucknow • Mumbai
Hyderabad • Jharkhand • Nagpur • Patna • Pune • Uttarakhand

OPHTHALMIC NURSING

ISBN: 978-81-239-0710-9

Copyright © AK Khurana

First Edition: 2000

Reprint: 2003, 2005, 2006, 2008, 2009, 2010, 2012, 2016, 2018, 2021, 2023, **2025**

Published by Satish Kumar Jain and produced by Varun Jain for

CBS Publishers & Distributors Pvt Ltd

4819/XI Prahlad Street, 24 Ansari Road, Daryaganj, New Delhi 110 002, India

Ph: 011-23289259, 23266861, 23266867   Website: www.cbspd.com

Fax: 011-23243014   e-mail: delhi@cbspd.com

Corporate Office: 204 FIE, Industrial Area, Patparganj, Delhi 110 092

Ph: 011-4934 4934   Fax: 011-4934 4935   e-mail: publishing@cbspd.com; publicity@cbspd.com

Branches

- **Bengaluru:** Seema House 2975, 17th Cross, KR Road, Banasankari 2nd Stage, Bengaluru 560 070, Karnataka, India
  Ph: +91-80-26771678/79   Fax: +91-80-26771680   e-mail: bangalore@cbspd.com
- **Chennai:** 7, Subbaraya Street, Shenoy Nagar, Chennai 600 030, Tamil Nadu, India
  Ph: +91-44-26680620, 26681266   Fax: +91-44-42032115   e-mail: chennai@cbspd.com
- **Kochi:** 42/1325, 1326, Power House Road, Opp KSEB, Power House, Ernakulam, Kochi 682 018, India
  Ph: +91-484-4059061–65   Fax: +91-484-4059065   e-mail: kochi@cbspd.com
- **Kolkata:** 147, Hind Ceramics Compound, 1st Floor, Nilgunj Road, Belghoria, Kolkata 700 056, West Bengal, India
  Ph: +91-33-25633055–56   e-mail: kolkata@cbspd.com
- **Lucknow:** Basement, Khushnuma Complex, 7-Meerabai Marg (behind Jawahar Bhawan), Lucknow 226 001, India
  Ph: +91-522-4000032   e-mail: tiwari.lucknow@cbspd.com
- **Mumbai:** PWD Shed. Gala no. 25/26, Ramchandra Bhatt Marg, Next to JJ Hospital Gate no. 2, Opp. Union Bank of India, Noorbaug Mumbai 400 009, Maharashtra, India
  Ph: +91-22-66661880/89   e-mail: mumbai@cbspd.com

Representatives

- **Hyderabad** 0-9885175004
- **Jharkhand** 0-9811541605
- **Nagpur** 0-9421945513
- **Patna** 0-9334159340
- **Pune** 0-9623451994
- **Uttarakhand** 0-9716462459

Printed at SRK Graphics, Delhi, India

Dedicated

- To nursing students and teachers for their service to suffering humans
- To my children, Aruj and Arushi, for their patience
- To my wife, Dr. Indu, for her understanding and encouragement
- To my parents and teachers for their blessings

Foreword

It is my pleasure to write the foreword for the book *'Ophthalmic Nursing'* by Dr. A. K. Khurana, who is an experienced teacher and has six other successful books on ophthalmology to his credit. This book is the result of his keen interest in improving the nursing care of ophthalmic patients.

The book has been organized into eighteen chapters. First chapter gives a brief account of the anatomy and physiology of eye which is essential to understand the eye diseases. In second chapter *'Role of a Nurse in Care of Ophthalmic Patients'* has been discussed in detail. Next fifteen chapters have been devoted to *'Diseases of the Eye'* in a concise way with an emphasis on nursing care, and the last chapter is on *'Community Ophthalmology'*. The book is written in a point-to-point stepwise pattern which will help the students to easily understand, retain and reproduce the subject matter.

Ophthalmic Nursing usually forms a section in most of the textbooks on *Medical-Surgical Nursing*. A separate book on this topic is a welcome addition to the shelf of 'Nursing Books'. Perhaps, it may be the first venture of its kind from India. I am sure this book will not only be useful for the nursing students but will also serve as a handbook and a life-long companion to the nursing professionals.

I am confident the book will fulfill its aim of raising the standard of nursing care of ophthalmic patients. I compliment the author for his maiden venture and wish him every success.

Shashi Sood
M.Sc. (Nursing)
Principal, School of Nursing
Postgraduate Institute of Medical Sciences
Rohtak - 124001

Preface

Ophthalmic nursing needs a specialized kind of skill and understanding. It combines principles of both medical and surgical nursing care. To learn the art of nursing care of ophthalmic patients, the nurses need to be familiar with the common diseases of the eye, which have been covered concisely in this book. An attempt has been made to describe the role of a nurse in the care of ophthalmic patients in a comprehensive and practically oriented manner. To understand diseases of the eye and principles of ophthalmic nursing the book begins with a working knowledge of anatomy and physiology of the eye.

This book is primarily intended for use by the students undertaking a nursing course and the nurses engaged in the care of eye patients. It may also be helpful to nurse-tutors, ward sisters and all those involved in teaching nurses in this speciality.

I record my sense of indebtness and gratitude to Mrs. Veeran Wanti, Nursing Superintendent and Miss Shashi Sood, Principal and other staff members of School of Nursing, Pt. B.D. Sharma Postgraduate Institute of Medical Sciences, Rohtak for their encouragement and valuable suggestions in completing this task. I acknowledge the timely help rendered by Dr. Vikas Thukral. I am thankful to Dr. R.C. Nagpal, Prof. and Head, Deptt. of Ophthalmology and Prof. S.B. Siwach, Director, PGIMS, Rohtak for providing a working atmosphere.

It is a special pleasure to acknowlege the most assured co-operation of Mr. Mahesh Gupta and M/s CBS Publishers & Distributors in general, and Mr. S. K. Jain, Managing Director and Mr. V. K. Jain, Production Director in particular. It is my proud previliage to admire my wife Dr. Indu Khurana. Assoc. Prof. of Physiology, PGIMS, Rohtak, who has always inspired and encouraged me for my academic pursuits.

Finally, despite best efforts, ventures of this kind are not likely to be free of ambiguities, some inaccuracies, human errors and typographic mistakes. Therefore, a feedback and active criticism from the students and teaching staff of nursing schools will be of utmost help in improving second edition of the book.

A. K. Khurana

Contents

1

Anatomy and
Physiology of the Eye

INTRODUCTION

Ophthalmic nursing needs a special kind of skill and understanding. To learn the art of nursing care of ophthalmic patients, the nurses need to be well versed with the common diseases of the eye. And to understand the eye diseases, a working knowledge of the anatomy and physiology of the eye is almost mandatory.

There are two eyeballs, each being suspended by *extraocular muscles* and fascial sheaths in a quadrilateral pyramid-shaped bony cavity called *orbit*. Each eye is protected anteriorly by two shutters called the *eyelids*. The anterior part of the sclera and posterior surface of the eyelids is lined by a thin membrane called *conjunctiva*. For smooth functioning, the cornea and conjunctiva are to be kept moist by tears, which are produced by the lacrimal gland and drained by lacrimal passages, which together form the *lacrimal apparatus*. The eyelids, the eyebrows, the conjunctiva and lacrimal apparatus are collectively known as the *appendages of the eye*.

A brief account of anatomy of the eyeball and its related structures is given below.

THE EYEBALL (Fig. 1.1)

Each eyeball is a cystic structure kept distended by the pressure inside it.

DIMENSIONS OF AN ADULT EYEBALL

Anteroposterior diameter	: 24 mm
Horizontal (transverse) diameter	: 23.5 mm
Vertical diameter	: 23 mm
Circumference	: 75 mm
Volume	: 6.5 ml
Weight	: 7 gm

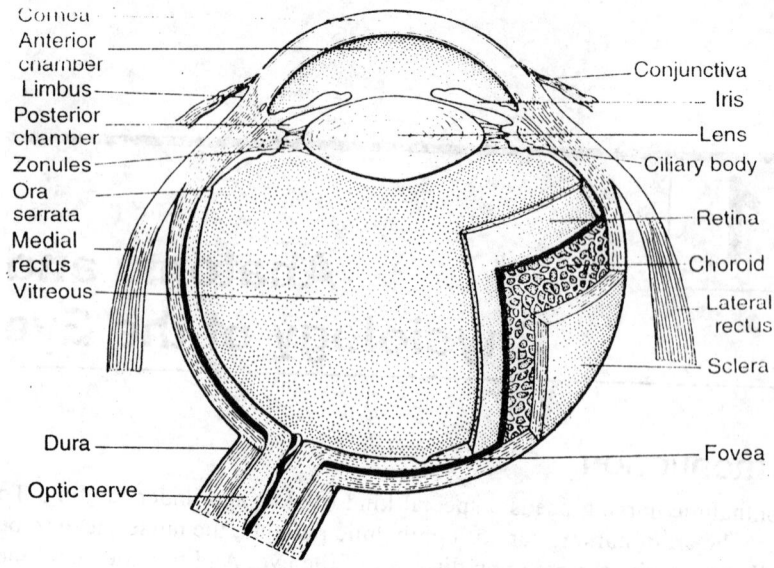

Fig. 1.1. Gross anatomy of the eyeball.

COATS OF THE EYEBALL

The eyeball comprises three coats; outer (fibrous coat), middle (vascular coat) and inner (nervous coat).

1. The outer fibrous coat (Fig. 1.1)

It is a dense strong wall which protects the intraocular contents. Anterior one-sixth of the fibrous coat is transparent and is called cornea. The posterior 5/6th opaque part is called sclera. Junction of the cornea and sclera is called limbus.

Cornea

The cornea is a transparent, avascular, watchglass like structure with a smooth shining surface. The average diameter of the cornea is 11-12 mm. Its thickness in the central part is 0.52 mm and in the peripheral part 0.67 mm. Histologically, cornea consists of following five layers (Fig. 1.2) :

1. *Epithelium.* It is of stratified squamous type and consists of 5-6 layers of cells.
2. *Bowman's membrane.* It consists of a cellular mass of condensed collagen fibrils. It does not regenerate when damaged.
3. *Stroma (substantia propria).* It forms 90% of corneal thickness. It mainly consists of regularly arranged collagen fibrils (lamellae)

Plate I

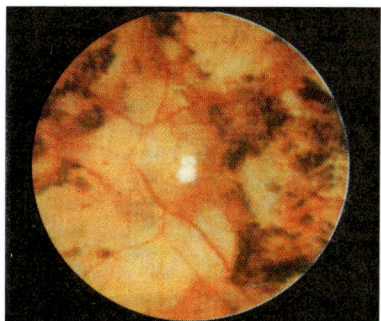

Pl. I.1. Myopic chorioretinal degeneration.

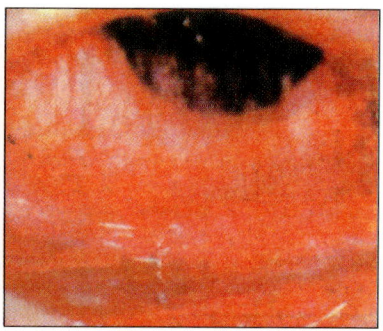

Pl. I.2. Acute bacterial conjunctivitis.

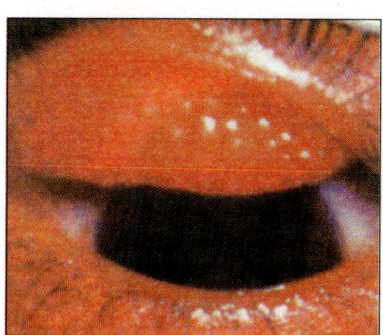

Pl. I.3. Trachomatous inflammation follicular (TF).

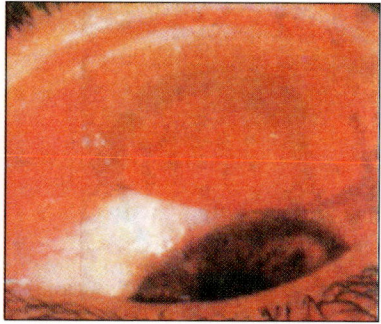

Pl. I.4. Trachomatous inflammation intense (TI).

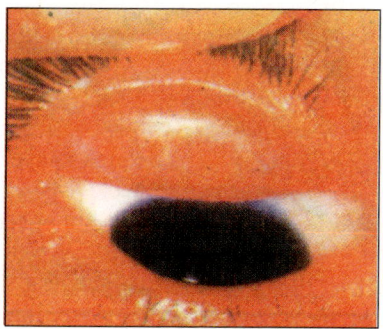

Pl. I.5. Trachomatous scarring (TS).

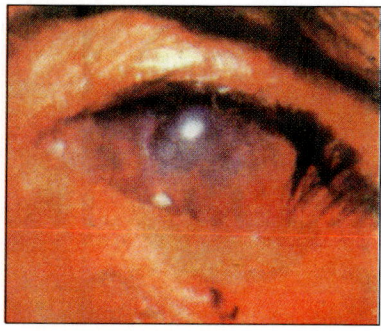

Pl. I.6. Trachomatous trichiasis (TT).

Plate II

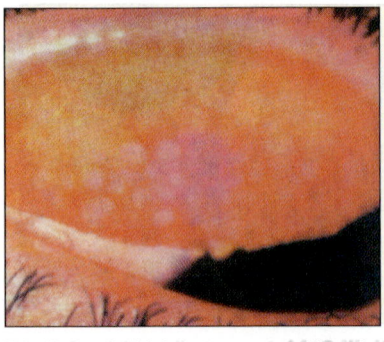

Pl. II.1. Cobble stone papillae in palpebral spring catarrh.

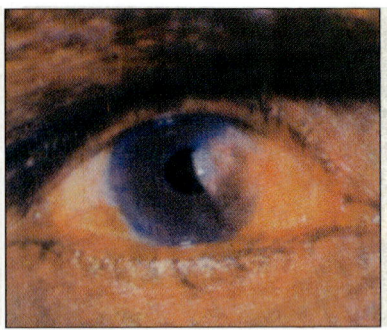

Pl. II.2. Pterygium.

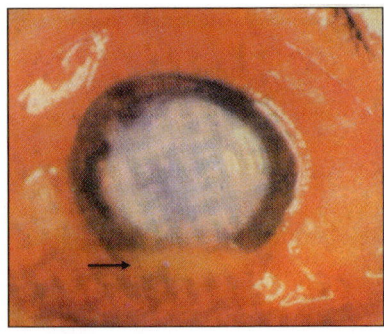
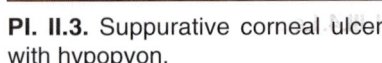

Pl. II.3. Suppurative corneal ulcer with hypopyon.

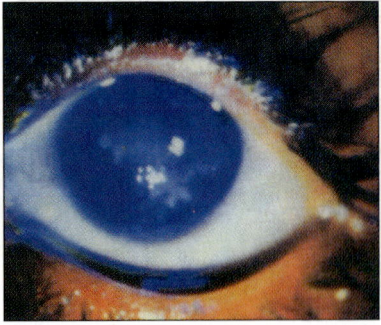

Pl. II.4. Dendritic corneal ulcer.

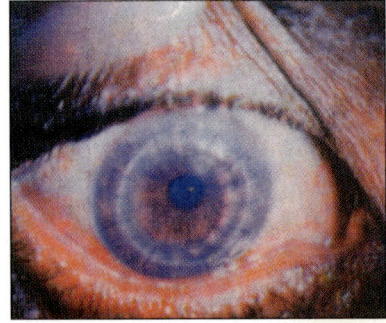

Pl. II.5. Keratoplasty with interrupted sutures.

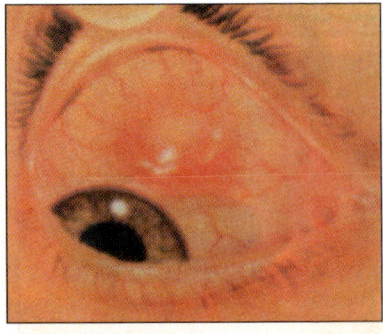

Pl. II.6. Nodular scleritis.

Plate III

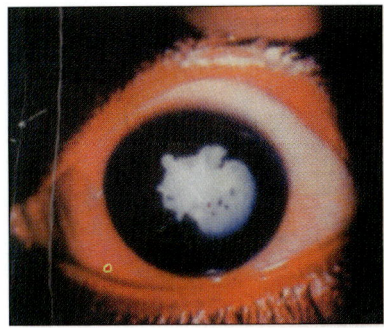

Pl. III.1. Iridocyclitis with posterior synechiae and complicated cataract.

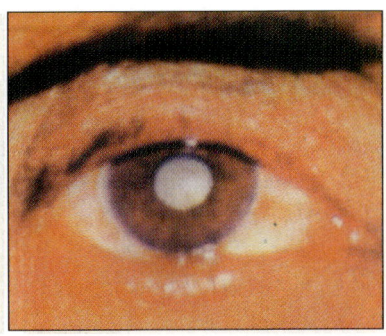

Pl. III.2. Mature senile cataract.

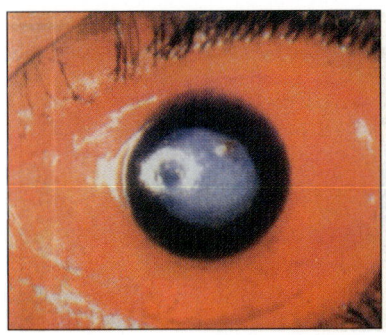

Pl. III.3. Phacomorphic glaucoma. Note ciliary congestion, pupil & intumescent lens.

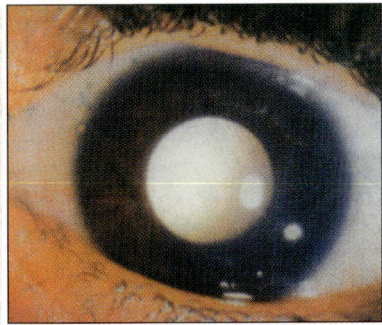

Pl. III.4. Leukocoria in retinoblastoma.

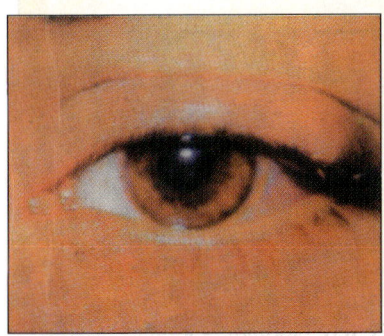

Pl. III.5. Style left upper lid.

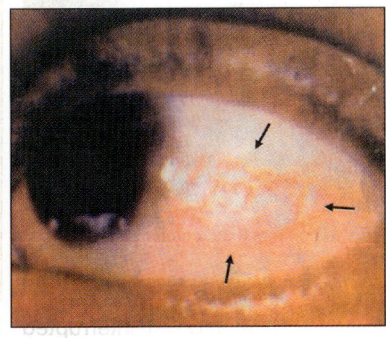

Pl. III.6. Bitot's spot.

embedded in ground substance. Among the lamellae are present keratocytes and few other cells.

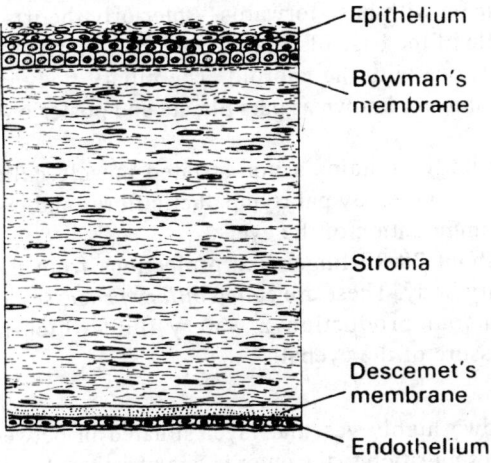

Fig. 1.2. Microscopic structure of the cornea.

4. *Descemet's membrane.* It is thin but strong homogenous elastic membrane. It is very resistant to chemical agents, trauma and pathological processes.

5. *Endothelium.* It consists of a single layer of flattened polygonal cells.

Nerve supply of cornea is purely sensory, derived from the ophthalmic division of the 5th cranial nerve.

Sclera

The sclera is a strong, opaque, white fibrous layer. It is a relatively avascular structure about 1 mm in thickness. It is pierced by nerves and vessels entering in the eyeball. Histologically, sclera consists of three layers : episcleral tissue, sclera proper and lamina fusca.

2. The middle vascular coat (Fig. 1.1)

The middle vascular coat also known as uveal tract, from anterior to posterior, can be divided into three parts - iris, ciliary body and choroid. The blood supply of uveal tract is derived from the short posterior ciliary arteries, long posterior ciliary arteries and anterior ciliary arteries.

Iris

It is a coloured, circular diaphragm with a central aperture of 3-4 mm in size known as pupil. The pupil regulates the light reaching the retina. The pupil constricts and dilates by the contraction of sphincter pupillae and dilator pupillae muscle of the iris, respectively. The sphincter pupillae is supplied by the parasympathetic nerves while the dilator pupillae is supplied by the sympathetic nerves.

Ciliary body

The ciliary body is middle part of the uveal tract. In cut section it is triangular in shape with base forwards. Anteriorly the iris is attached to about the middle of the base of ciliary body. Posteriorly, the ciliary body becomes continuous with the choroid. The ciliary body can be divided into two parts - anterior known as pars plicata and posterior known as pars plana.

The ciliary body contains a non-striated muscle called the ciliary muscle which is supplied by parasympathetic fibres and takes part in the process of accommodation of the eye.

There are about 70-80 finger-like projections from the pars plicata part of the ciliary body. These are called *ciliary processes* and are the site of aqueous humour production - a watery fluid which maintains the intraocular pressure of the eyeball.

Choroid

It is a dark brown highly vascular layer situated in between sclera and retina. It supplies nutrition to the outer layers of retina. The inflammations of choroid invariably involve the overlying retina.

3. The inner nervous coat (Retina) (Fig. 1.3)

Retina, the innermost tunic of the eyeball, is a thin, delicate, transparent membrane. It is the most highly developed tissue of the eye. It is concerned with the visual functions.

Gross anatomy. Grossly, retina can be divided into optic disc, macula lutea and the peripheral retina.

Ora serrata is the anterior serrated termination of the retina.

Macula lutea (Yellow spot) is a comparatively dark area situated at the posterior pole temporal to the optic disc. Its central depressed area of 1.5 mm in diameter is called *fovea centralis,* which is the most sensitive part of the retina. Visual acuity is maximum in this part of retina.

Optic disc. It is a well-defined circular, pink coloured disc of 1.5 mm diameter. It has only nerve fibre layer, so it does not excite any visual response. It produces *blind spot* in the field of vision.

Structure (Fig. 1.4). Retina consists of ten layers, which from without inwards are as follows :

1. *Layer of pigment epithelium.* It is a single layer of hexagonal cells containing melanin pigments.
2. *Layer of rods and cones.* Rods and cones are end organs of vision and are also known as photoreceptors.
3. *External limiting membrane.* It is a thin fenestrated membrane.
4. *Outer nuclear layer.* It consists of nuclei of the rods and cones.
5. *Outer plexiform layer.* It consists of connections of axons of rods and cones with the dendrites of the bipolar cells.

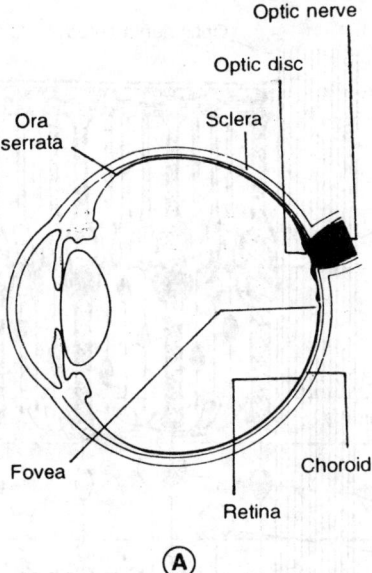

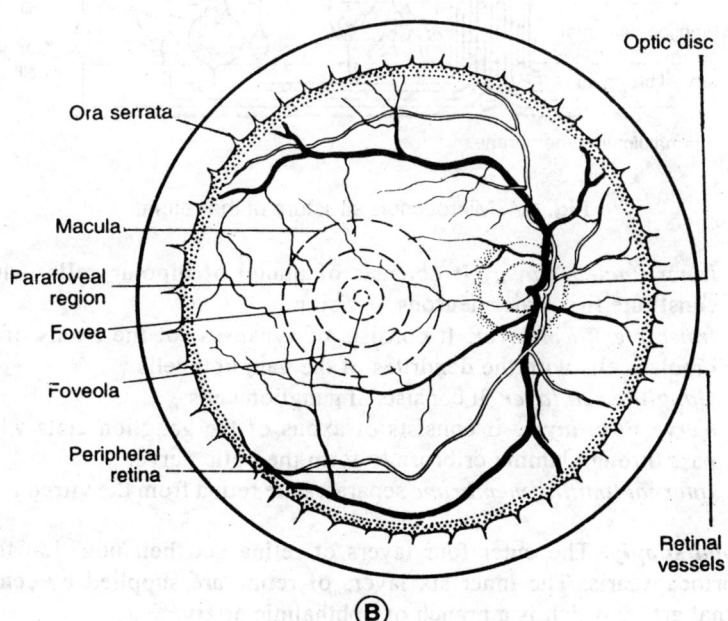

Fig. 1.3. Gross anatomy of the retina.

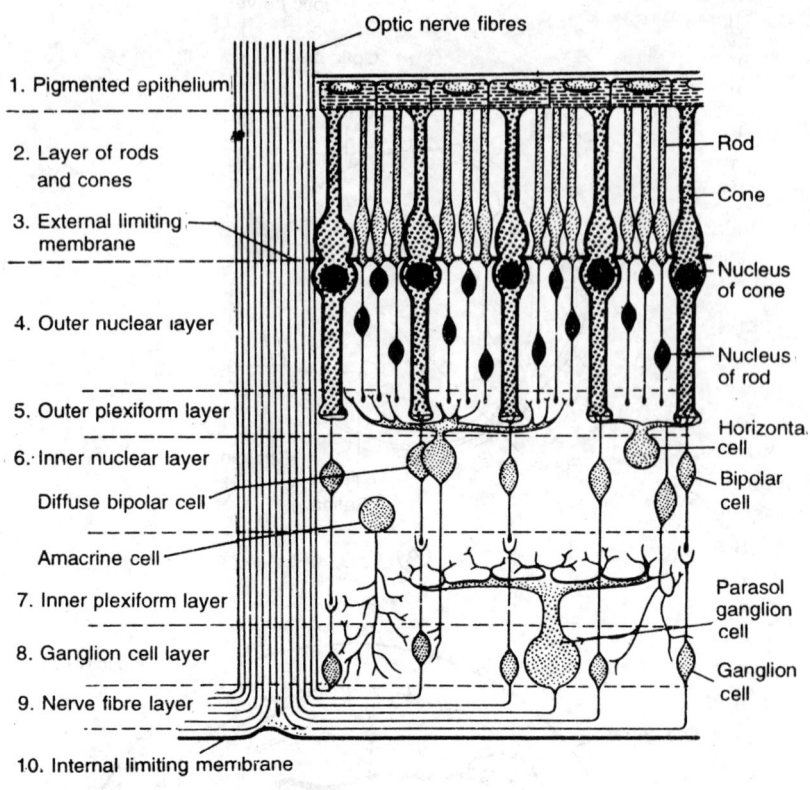

1. Pigmented epithelium
2. Layer of rods and cones
3. External limiting membrane
4. Outer nuclear layer
5. Outer plexiform layer
6. Inner nuclear layer
   Diffuse bipolar cell
   Amacrine cell
7. Inner plexiform layer
8. Ganglion cell layer
9. Nerve fibre layer
10. Internal limiting membrane

Optic nerve fibres
Rod
Cone
Nucleus of cone
Nucleus of rod
Horizontal cell
Bipolar cell
Parasol ganglion cell
Ganglion cell

Fig. 1.4. Microscopic structure of the retina.

6. *Inner nuclear layer.* It consists of nuclei of bipolar cells, which constitute first order neurons of vision.
7. *Inner plexiform layer.* It consists of synapses of the axons of the bipolar cells with the dendrites of the ganglion cells.
8. *Ganglion cell layer.* It consists of ganglion cells.
9. *Nerve fibre layer.* It consists of axons of the ganglion cells which pass through lamina cribrosa to form the optic nerve.
10. *Internal limiting membrane* separates the retina from the vitreous.

Blood supply. The outer four layers of retina get their nutrition from choriocapillaris. The inner six layers of retina are supplied by central retinal artery which is a branch of ophthalmic artery.

INTERIOR OF THE EYEBALL

Interior of the eyeball contains, from anterior to posterior, the aqueous humour, lens and vitreous.

Aqueous humour

It is a watery fluid present in the anterior and posterior chambers of the eyeball. *Anterior chamber* is the space bounded anteriorly by the back of cornea and posteriorly by the anterior surface of iris. *Posterior chamber* is the space between the front of crystalline lens and back of iris. Through pupil, anterior and posterior chambers communicate with each other.

Crystalline lens

The lens is a transparent, biconvex, crystalline structure placed between the iris and the vitreous. It is suspended from the ciliary body by the suspensory ligament or zonules of Zinn. Refractive power of the lens is about 15-16 D. Lens is elastic in nature and its power changes with accommodation. Elasticity of the lens gradually decreases with the age. It is a vascular structure and derives its nutrition from the aqueous humour.

Structure. It consists of (Fig. 1.5)

1. *Lens capsule* is a thin transparent structure enclosing the lens matter.
2. *The lenticular epithelium.* It is a single layer of cuboidal cells which lies deep to the anterior capsule.
3. *Lens fibres.* These form the main bulk of the lens and are arranged compactly as *nucleus* and *cortex* of the lens.

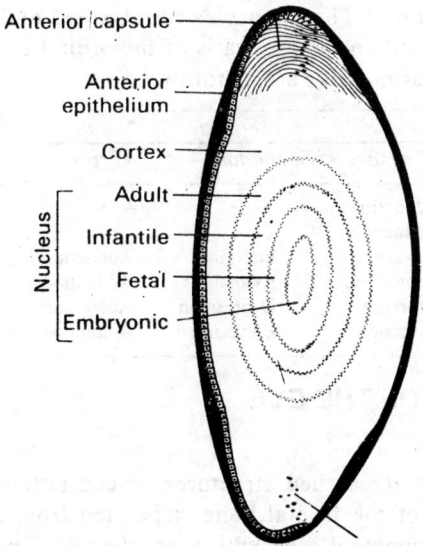

Fig. 1.5. Structure of the crystalline lens.

Vitreous humour

Vitreous humour is an inert, transparent, jelly-like structure that fills the posterior four-fifths of the cavity of eyeball. It serves the optical function. It consists of 90% water, some salts and mucoproteins.

EXTRAOCULAR MUSCLES (Fig. 1.6)

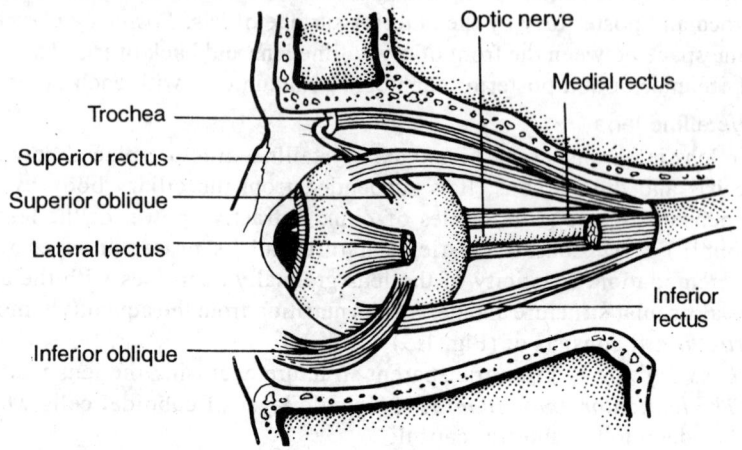

Fig. 1.6. Extraocular muscles.

A set of six extraocular muscles (4 recti and 2 obliques) control the movements of each eye. These muscles are attached to the outer coat of the eyeball at one end and to the walls of the orbital cavity at the other end. The extraocular muscles are as follows :

Muscle	Actions			Nerve
	Primary	*Secondary*	*Tertiary*	*Supply*
Medial rectus	Adduction	–	–	3rd N
Lateral rectus	Abduction	–	–	6th N
Superior rectus	Elevation	Intorsion	Adduction	3rd N
Inferior rectus	Depression	Extorsion	Adduction	3rd N
Superior oblique	Intorsion	Depression	Abduction	4th N
Inferior oblique	Extorsion	Elevation	Abduction	3rd N

APPENDAGES OF THE EYE

Eyebrows

The two eyebrows are arched structures placed horizontally over the superciliary ridge of the frontal bone, separated from each other by a smooth hairless prominent area known as glabella. The surface of the eyebrows is covered by hair which project obliquely from the skin and form an important part of the eyebrows. They protect the eyeball from sweat, dust and other foreign bodies.

Eyelids

The eyelids are mobile tissue curtains placed in front of the eyeballs. These act as shutters protecting the eyes from injuries and excessive light. These also perform an important function of spreading the tear film over the cornea and conjunctiva.

Eye lashes are short curved hair present on the lid margins (free edges of the eyelids).

Structure. From anterior to posterior the eyelid consists of following layers (Fig. 1.7)

1. *Skin.* It is elastic and very thin.
2. *Subcutaneous loose areolar tissue.*
3. *Layer of striated muscles.* It consists of orbicularis oculi muscle which closes the lids. In addition, the upper eyelid also contains levator palpebrae superioris muscle which raises the upper eyelids.

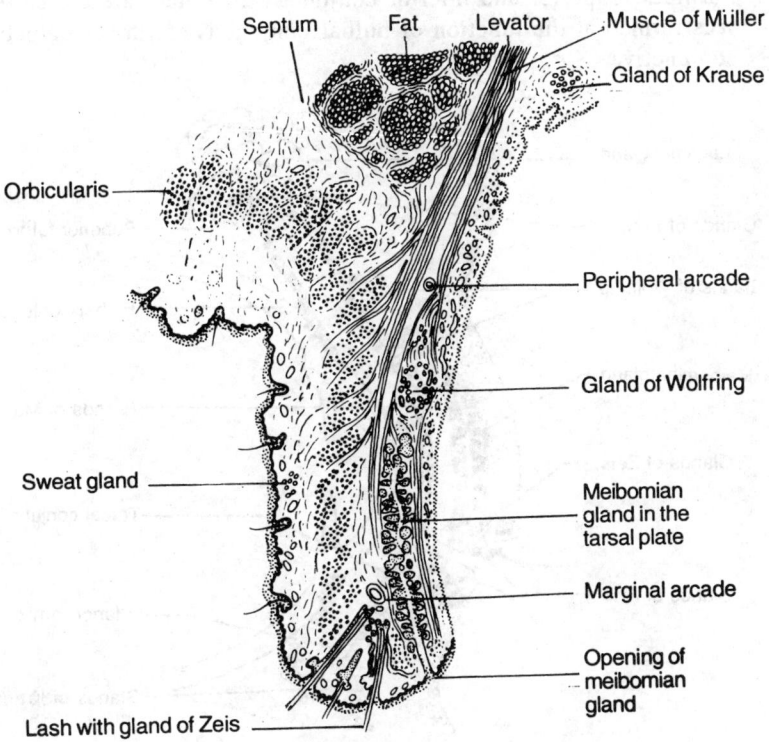

Fig. 1.7. Structure of the upper eyelid.

4. *Submuscular areolar tissue.* The nerves and vessels of the eyelids lie in this layer.
5. *Fibrous layer.* It is the framework of the lids and consists of two parts: the central *tarsal plate* and the peripheral septum orbitale.
6. *Layer of nonstriated muscle* fibres is formed by palpebral muscle of Muller.
7. *Conjunctiva.* The lids on their inner surface are lined by a thin mucous membrane called the palpebral conjunctiva.

Conjunctiva

The conjunctiva is a translucent mucous membrane which lines the posterior surface of the eyelids and anterior aspect of the eyeball upto limbus.

Parts. Conjunctiva consists of following parts (Fig. 1.8) :
1. *Palpebral conjunctiva* lines the posterior surface of the eyelids.
2. *Bulbar conjunctiva* covers the anterior part of eyeball upto the limbus.
3. *Fornices.* Superior and inferior conjunctival fornices are the cul-de-sacs formed at the junction of bulbar conjunctiva with the palpebral conjunctiva.

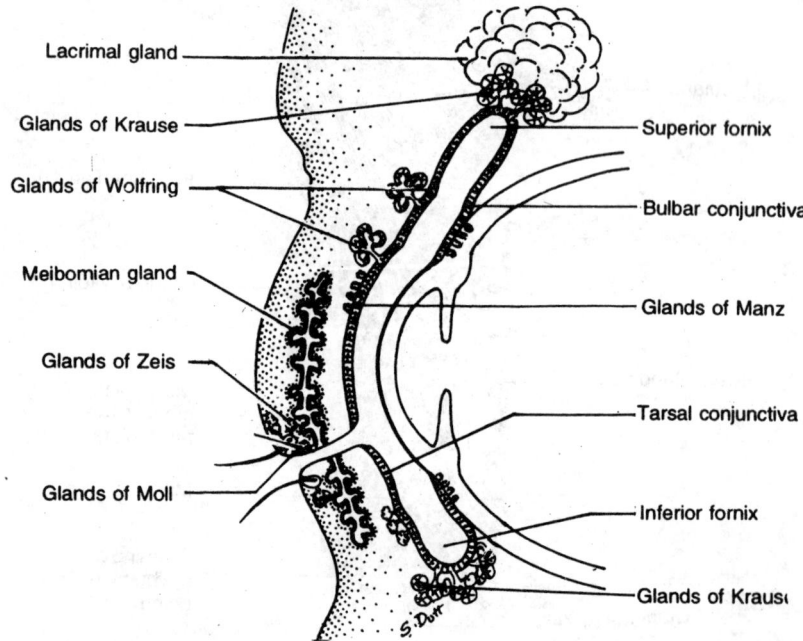

Fig. 1.8. Parts of conjunctiva and conjunctival glands.

4. *Plica semilunaris* is a pinkish crescentric fold of conjunctiva present in the medial canthus.

Lacrimal apparatus

The lacrimal apparatus (Fig. 1.9) comprises the structures concerned with the formation (main lacrimal gland and accessary lacrimal glands) and drainage (lacrimal passages: puncta, canaliculi, lacrimal sac and nasolacrimal duct) of tears.

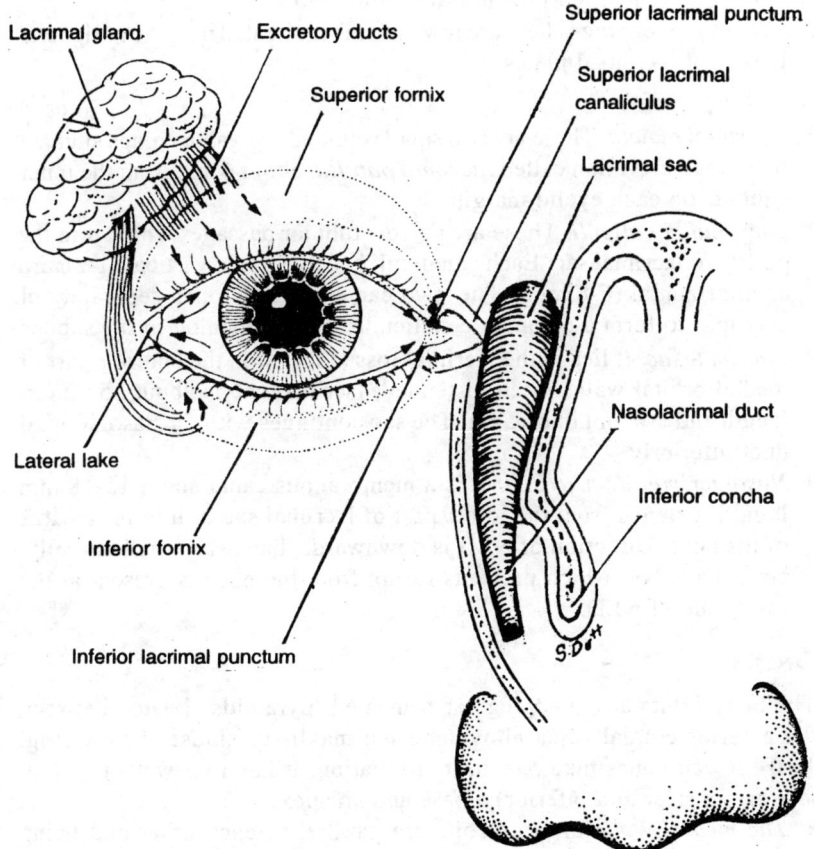

Fig. 1.9. The lacrimal apparatus.

Main lacrimal gland

The main lacrimal gland is situated at the upper and outer angle of the orbit, in a depression known as the fossa for the lacrimal gland. It consists of an upper orbital and a lower palpebral part. Each gland is about the size and shape of an almond. It is composed of secretory epithelial cells.

The ducts of lacrimal gland which are about 12 in number open in the superior fornix. The gland secretes tears composed of water, salt and lysozyme (a bactericidal enzyme).

Accessory lacrimal glands

1. *Glands of Krause.* These are microscopic glands situated beneath the palpebral conjunctiva between fornix and edge of the tarsal plate. There are about 42 in upperlid and 6-8 in lower lid.
2. *Glands of Wolfring.* There are few in number situated near the peripheral border of the tarsal plates.

Lacrimal passages

1. *Lacrimal puncta.* These are two small rounded or oval openings situated on a small elevation called *lacrimal papilla,* about 6 mm from the inner canthus on each eyelid margin.
2. *Lacrimal canaliculi.* These are narrow tubular passages which join the puncta to lacrimal sac. Each canaliculi has two parts: vertical (1-2 mm) and horizontal (6-8 mm). The two canaliculi may open separately or may join to form a common canaliculus before opening in the sac.
3. *Lacrimal sac.* It lies in the lacrimal fossa located in the anterior part of medial orbital wall. When distended, lacrimal sac is about 15 mm in length and 5-6 mm in breadth. The sac continues with the nasolacrimal duct inferiorly.
4. *Nasolacrimal duct (NLD).* It is a membranous canal about 15-18 mm long. It extends from the lower part of lacrimal sac to inferior meatus of the nose. Direction of NLD is downwards, backwards and laterally. Hasner's valve, which prevents reflux from the nose, is present at the lower end of NLD.

ORBIT

The bony orbits are quadrangular truncated pyramids situated between the anterior cranial fossa above and the maxillary sinuses below (Fig. 1.10). Seven bones take part in its formation. It has four walls (medial, lateral, superior and inferior), a base and an apex.

- *The medial walls* of two orbits are parallel to each other and being thinnest are frequently fractured during orbital injuries. Thinness of the medial wall also accounts for ethmoiditis being the commonest cause of orbital cellulitis.
- *The inferior wall (floor)* is triangular in shape and being quite thin is commonly involved in blow-out fractures.
- *The lateral wall* is triangular in shape and thickest, particularly at the orbital margin. It covers only posterior half of the eyeball.
- *The roof* of the orbit is mainly formed by the orbital plate of frontal bone.

- *The orbital apex* is the posterior end of the orbit. Here the four orbital walls converge. It has two orifices the *optic canal* which transmits optic nerve and ophthalmic artery and the superior orbital fissure which transmits a number of nerves, arteries and veins.

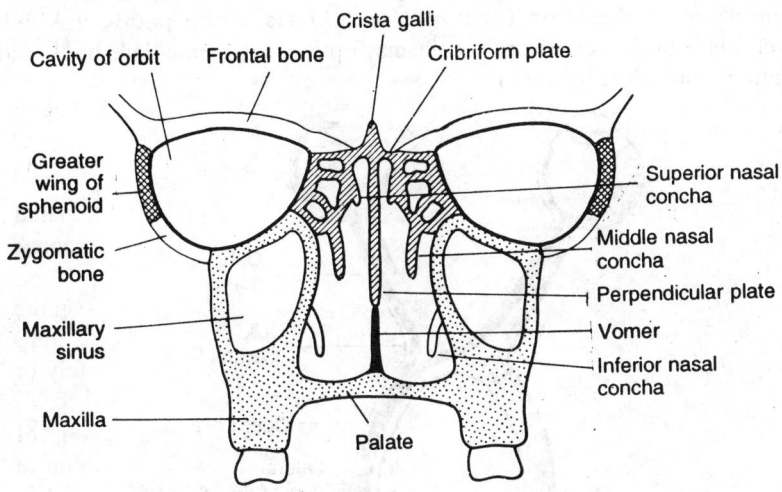

Fig. 1.10. Schematic coronal section through the orbits and nasal cavity.

Contents of the orbit

The volume of each orbit is about 30 cc. Approximately one-fifth of it is occupied by the eyeball. Other contents of the orbit include part of optic nerve, extraocular muscles, orbital fascia, lacrimal gland, lacrimal sac, ophthalmic artery and its branches, third, fourth and sixth cranial nerves, ophthalmic and maxillary divisions of the fifth cranial nerve, sympathetic nerves and orbital fat.

Surgical spaces in the orbit

There are four surgical spaces in the orbit. These are of clinical importance as the inflammatory process remains localized in any one of them and each space may be opened separately.

1. *Subperiosteal space.* It is a potential space which lies between bone and the periorbita.
2. *Peripheral space.* It is a continuous circular space which lies between the periorbita and the four rectus muscles with their intermuscular septa.
3. *Central space* or the retrobulbar space is a cone-shaped space behind the eyeball, enclosed by the four rectus muscles with their inter-muscular septa. It is also called muscle cone.
4. *Tenon's space.* It is a potential space around the eyeball between the Tenon's capsule and the sclera. Tenon's capsule is the fascia which

surrounds the globe of the eye. It separates the eyeball from the orbital fat. The extraocular muscles pierce this capsule.

VISUAL PATHWAY

Each eyeball acts as a camera; it perceives the images and relays the sensations to the brain (occipital cortex) via visual pathway which comprises optic nerve, optic chiasma, optic tract, geniculate body and optic radiations (Fig. 1.11).

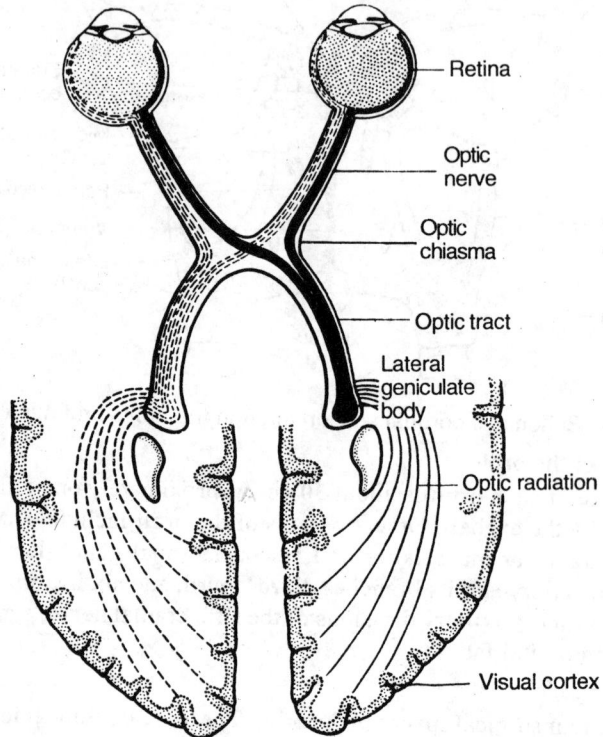

Retina

Optic nerve

Optic chiasma

Optic tract

Lateral geniculate body

Optic radiation

Visual cortex

Fig. 1.11. Gross anatomy of the visual pathways.

1. *Optic nerve.* Each optic nerve (second cranial nerve) starts from the optic disc and extends upto the optic chiasma. It is the continuation backward of the nerve fibre layer of retina, which consists of the axons of the ganglion cells.

   The optic nerve is about 47-50 mm in length and can be divided into four parts : intraocular (1 mm), intraorbital (30 mm), intracanalicular (6-9 mm) and intracranial (10 mm). The optic nerve is covered by all the three meningeal sheaths of the brain viz., pia mater, arachnoid and dura.

2. *Optic chiasma.* It is a flattened structure lying above the pituitary fossa. Fibres originating from the nasal halves of the retina decussate at the chiasma.

3. *Optic tracts.* These are cylindrical bundles of nerve fibres which originate from the posterolateral angle of the chiasma and outwards and backwards to end in the lateral geniculate bodies. They consist of the temporal fibres of the same side and the nasal fibres of the opposite side.

4. *Lateral geniculate bodies:* These are oval structures situated at the posterior termination of the optic tracts. The fibres of the optic tracts end in the lateral geniculate bodies and nerve fibres of the optic radiations originate from them.

5. *Optic radiations.* These extend from the lateral geniculate bodies to the visual cortex.

6. *Visual cortex.* It is located on the medial aspect of the occipital lobe, above and below the calcarine fissure. It is subdivided into the visuo-sensory area (striate area 17) that receives the fibres of the radiations, and the surrounding visuo-psychic area (peristriate area 18 and parastriate area 19).

PHYSIOLOGY OF THE EYE

Funtion of the eyes is to provide sense of sight (vision), which is the choicest gift from the Almighty to humans and other animals. The eyeballs are able to perform their function with the help of following physiological activities.

1. Maintenance of clear media of the eye.
2. Maintenance of normal intraocular pressure (See page 141)
3. Neurophysiology of vision.
4. Mechanism of sight.
5. Physiology of binocular vision.

MAINTENANCE OF CLEAR MEDIA OF THE EYE

The main factor responsible for transparency of the refractive media of the eye is their avascularity. The structures forming refractive media of the eye from anterior to posterior are as below :

1. Tear film. It keeps the cornea moist and provides oxygen and nutrients. Structure of tear film is described on page 181.

2. Cornea. It forms the main refracting medium of the eye. Corneal transparency is the result of peculiar arrangement of its lamellae, avascularity and relative state of dehydration, which is maintained by barrier effects of epithelium and endothelium and an active pump mechanism present in the endothelial cells.

3. *Aqueous humour.* It is a clear watery fluid filling the anterior chamber and posterior chamber of the eye. In addition to maintaining intraocular pressure it also provides nutrients to the cornea and crystalline lens. For details see page 141

4. *Crystalline lens.* It is a biconvex lens which has been provided with a unique mechanism of changing its power (*accommodation*). Due to this characteristic it helps in sharp focusing of the images of the objects present at varying distances from the eye.

5. *Vitreous humour.* It is clear jelly-like material which in addition to being a refractive medium also helps in maintaining the shape of the eyeball.

NEUROPHYSIOLOGY OF VISION

Neurophysiology of vision is a complex phenomenon which is still poorly understood. The main mechanisms concerned with vision are as follows:

1. Initiation and transmission of visual sensation

Light falling upon the retina initiates photochemical changes in the visual pigments of rod and cone cells. The photochemical reaction initiates the visual sensation in the form of changes in electrical potential which are transmitted through the bipolar cells to the ganglion cells and along the fibres of the optic nerve to the brain.

2. Visual perception

It is a complex integration of following senses:
  i. *The light sense.* It is awareness of presence of light.
  ii. *The form sense.* It is the ability to discriminate between the shapes of the objects. Cones play a major role in this faculty.
  iii. *The contrast sense.* It is the ability of the eye to perceive slight changes in the luminance between regions which are not separated by definite borders.
  iv. *The colour sense.* It is the ability of the eye to discriminate between different colours.

MECHANISM OF SIGHT

As described on page 72 the functioining of the eye as an optical instrument can be compared with a camera (Fig. 1.12) as below :
- *Eyelids* act as shutter of the camera.
- *Cornea and crystalline lens* act as focusing system of the camera.
- *Iris* acts as diaphragm which regulates the size of the aperture (*pupil*) and therefore the amount of light entering the eye.
- *Choroid* helps in forming the darkened interior of the camera.
- *Retina* acts as light sensitive plate or film on which image is formed.

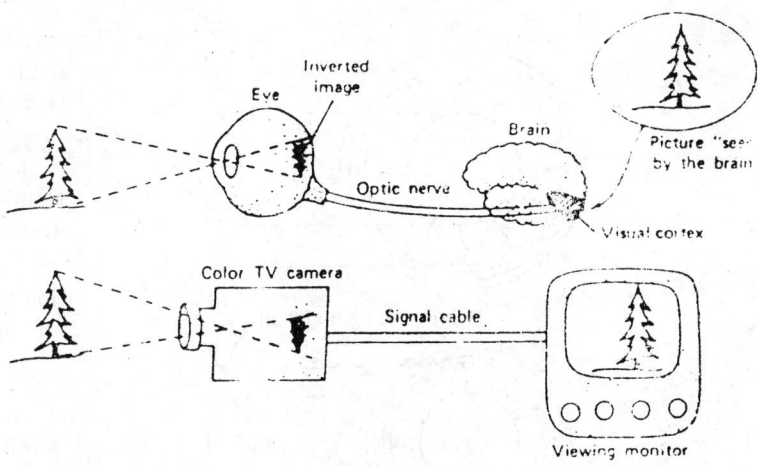

Fig. 1.12. The sense of sight is in many ways similar to a closed circuit colour TV system. It is superior in all respects except ease of replacement.

The optic nerve and its connections convey the details of the image to the occipital region of the cerebral cortex where they are processed before reaching consciousness.

ACCOMMODATION

As we know that in an emmetropic eye, parallel rays of light coming from infinity are brought to focus on the retina, with accommodation being at rest. However, our eyes have been provided with a unique mechanism by which we can even focus the diverging rays coming from a near object on the retina in a bid to see clearly (Fig. 1.13). This mechanism is called *accommodation.* In it there occurs increase in the power of crystalline lens due to increase in the curvature of its surfaces (Fig. 1.14).

At rest the radius of curvature of the anterior surface of the lens is 10 mm and that of posterior surface is 6 mm. In accommodation, the curvature of

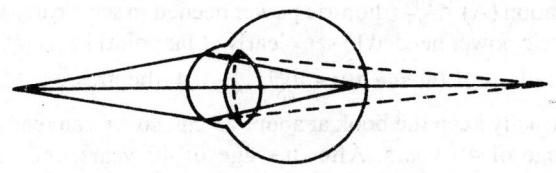

Fig. 1.13. Effect of accommodation on divergent rays entering the eye.

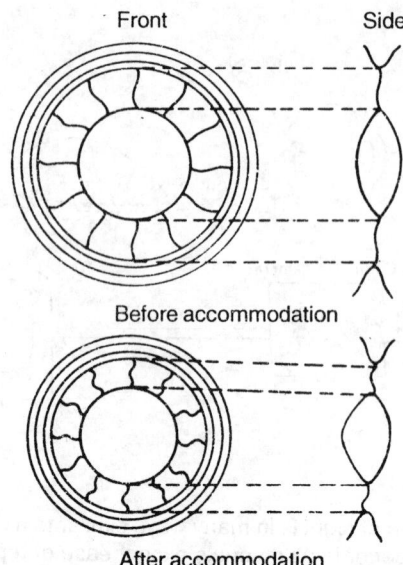

Fig. 1.14. Changes in the ciliary body ring, zonules and shape of lens during accommodation.

the posterior surface remains almost the same, but the anterior surface changes, so that in strong accommodation its radius of curvature becomes 6 mm.

The nearest point at which small objects can be seen clearly is called *near point* or *punctum proximum* and the distant (farthest) point is called *far point* or *punctum remotum*. The distance between the near point and the far point is called the *range of accommodation*. The difference between the dioptric power needed to focus at near point (P) and far point (R) is called *amplitude of accommodation* (A). Thus A = P − R.

Far point and near point of the eye vary with the static refraction of the eye. In hypermetropic eye far point is virtual and lies behind the eye while in myopic eye it is real and lies in front of the eye (Fig. 1.15).

In an emmetropic eye, far point is infinity and near point varies with age (being about 7 cm at the age of 10 years, 25 cm at the age of 40 years and 33 cm at the age of 45 years). Therefore, at the age of 10 years, amplitude of accommodation (A) = $\frac{100}{25}$ (dioptric power needed to see clearly at near point) - 1/∞ (dioptric power needed to see clearly at far point) i.e. A (at age 10) = 14 dioptres; similarly A (at age 40) = $\frac{100}{25} - \frac{1}{\infty}$ = 4 dioptres.

Since, we usually keep the book at about 25 cm, so we can read comfortably up to the age of 40 years. After the age of 40 years, the near point of accommodation recedes beyond the normal reading or working range. *This condition of failing near vision due to age-related decrease in the amplitude of accommodation or increase in punctum proximum is called presbyopia.*

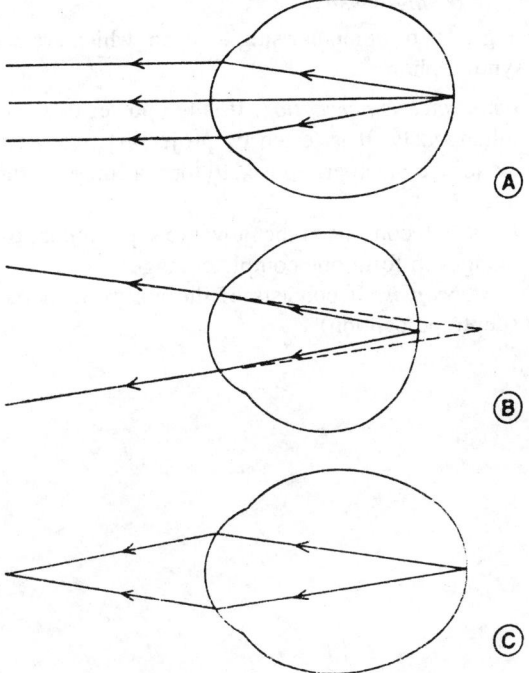

Fig. 1.15. Far point in emmetropic eye (A), hypermetropic eye (B), and myopic eye (C).

BINOCULAR SINGLE VISION

When a normal individual fixes his visual attention on an object of regard, the image is formed on the fovea of both the eyes separately; but the individual perceives a single image. This state is called binocular single vision. It is a conditioned reflex which is not present since birth but is acquired during first 6 months and is completed during first few years. The process of its development is complex and partially understood.

Prerequisites for development of binocular single vision

1. *Straight eyes* starting from the neonatal period with precise coordination for all directions of gaze (motor mechanism).
2. *Reasonably clear vision* in both eyes so that similar images are presented to each retina (sensory mechanism).
3. *Ability of visual cortex* to promote binocular single vision (mental process). Therefore, pathologic states disturbing any of the above mechanisms during the first few years of life will hinder the development of binocular single vision and may cause squint.

Grades of binocular single vision

There are three grades of binocuiar single vision, which are best tested with the help of a synoptophore.

- *Grade I—Simultaneous perception.* It is the power to see two dissimilar objects simultaneously. It is tested by projecting two dissimilar objects (which can be joined or superimposed to form a complete picture) in front of the two eyes.
- *Grade II—Fusion.* It consists of the power to superimpose two incomplete but similar images to form one complete image.
- *Grade III— Stereopsis.* It consists of the ability to perceive the third dimension (depth perception).

2

Role of a Nurse in Care of Ophthalmic Patients

INTRODUCTION

Ophthalmology is a branch of medical sciences which deals with the diseases of the eyeball and its related ocular structures. Present day ophthalmology is very much advanced and highly specialized. To keep pace with the modern advances in medical sciences, not only doctors, but nurses also need a specialized training. In fact, ophthalmic nursing has become a specialized training in the developed countries to be undertaken after the general nursing course. However, in the developing countries, still a general nurse has to care for the ophthalmic patients. Therefore, it is mandatory that a student nurse should be adequately trained in ophthalmic nursing. Undoubtedly, a student nurse before entering the specialized field of ophthalmology, undergoes a sufficient experience in general nursing. However, she should understand that care of an ophthalmic patient needs a special kind of skill and understanding.

This chapter deals with the basic principles of ophthalmic nursing. The specific nursing care needed by an individual suffering from particular diseases is described along with the disease process concerned in the ensuing chapters.

In general, role of a nurse in ophthalmology can be discussed under following sections :

1. *Clinical ocular examination and diagnostic techniques*
2. *Nursing procedures*
   i. Instillation of eye drops and eye ointments.
   ii. Cleaning/swabbing the eyelids.
   iii. Hot and cold eye compresses.
   iv. Irrigation of the eyes
   v. Removal, insertion and care of an artificial eye
3. *Nursing care of eye patients*
   i. General guidelines for nursing care of ophthalmic patients.

ii. Nursing care of the non-seeing patient.
iii. Preoperative nursing care.
iv. Postoperative nursing care
v. Role of a nurse in ophthalmic operation theatre
vi. Role of a nurse in mobile eye clinics and eye camps.
vii. Nurse as a community eye health worker (see page 203)

CLINICAL OCULAR EXAMINATION AND DIAGNOSTIC TECHNIQUES

A staff nurse working in the department of ophthalmology has to help the ophthalmologist during clinical ocular examination and while performing the various diagnostic techniques. So, she needs to be familiar with various examination techniques and the equipments required for various diagnostic techniques.

OCULAR EXAMINATION

I. TESTING OF VISUAL ACUITY

The nurse usually undertakes this task and it is necessary for her to become familiar with the various methods of estimating visual acuity, including those used when dealing with young children unable to read or with illiterate patients.

The visual acuity of each eye should be tested separately both for distance and near.

The distant visual acuity

The distant visual acuity in adults and school children is tested by using Snellen's test types (Fig. 2.1) or its equivalent viz. Landolt's C-chart or E-chart. In preschool children (below 3 years) isolated hand-tissue test or illiterate E-chart (Fig. 2.2) or pictorial vision charts (Fig. 2.3) may be used.

Procedure of testing visual acuity using Snellen's test types

Procedure of testing. For testing distant visual acuity, the patient is seated at a distance of 6 m from the Snellen's chart, so that the rays of light are practically parallel and the patient exerts minimal accommodation. The chart should be properly illuminated (not less than 20 ft candles). The patient is asked to read the chart with each eye separately and the visual acuity is recorded as a fraction, the numerator being the distance of the patient from the letters, and the denominator being the smallest letters accurately read.

When the patient is able to read up to 6 m line, the visual acuity is recorded as 6/6, which is normal. Similarly depending upon the smallest line which the patient can read from the distance of 6 m, his vision is recorded as 6/9, 6/12, 6/18, 6/24, 6/36 and 6/60, respectively. If he cannot see the top line from 6 m, he is asked to slowly walk towards the chart till he can read the top line. Depending upon the distance at which he can read the top line, his vision is recorded as 5/60, 4/60, 3/60, 2/60 and 1/60, respectively.

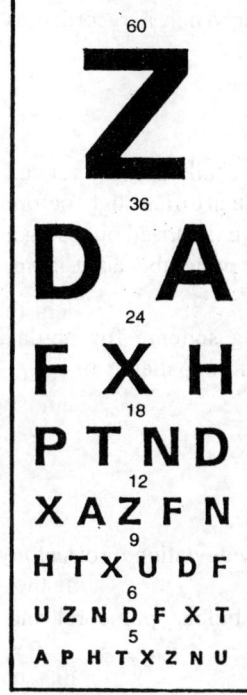

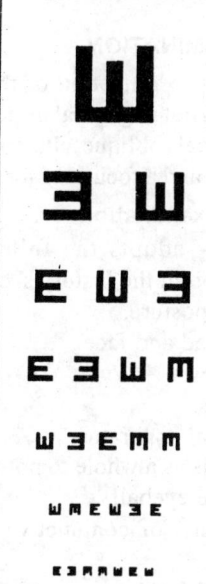

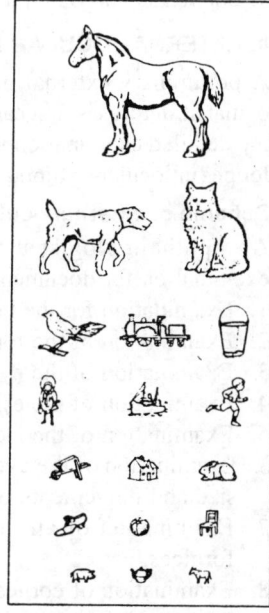

Fig. 2.1. Snellen's test types.

Fig. 2.2. 'E' test types.

Fig. 2.3. Pictorial vision chart.

If the patient is unable to read the top line even from 1 m, he is asked to count fingers (CF) of the examiner. His vision is recorded as CF-3', CF-2', CF-1' or CF close to face, depending upon the distance at which the patient is able to count fingers. When the patient fails to count fingers, the examiner moves his hand close to the patient's face. If he can appreciate the hand movements (HM), visual acuity is recorded as HM +ve. When the patient cannot distinguish the hand movements, the examiner notes whether the patient can perceive light (PL) or not. If yes, vision is recorded as PL +ve and if not it is recorded as PL –ve.

Visual acuity for near

Near vision is tested by asking the patient to read the near vision chart , kept at a distance of 35 cm in good illumination, with each eye separately. In near vision charts, a series of different sizes of printer type are arranged in increasing order and marked accordingly. Commonly used near vision charts are as follows:

1. *Jaeger's chart.* In this chart prints are marked from 1 to 7 and accordingly patient's acuity is labelled as J1 to J7 depending upon the print he can read.

2. *Roman test types.* According to this chart, the near vision is recorded as N5, N8, N10, N12 and N18 (Printer's point system).

3. *Snellen's near vision test types.*

II. EXTERNAL OCULAR EXAMINATION

A preliminary external ocular examination of the eyeballs and the related ocular structures is first carried out as general inspection in diffuse light before the detailed examination in focal (oblique) illumination is carried out using a loupe (uniocular or binocular) and a focussing torch or preferably a slit-lamp.

Scheme of external ocular examination

An ophthalmologist usually adopts the following scheme for ocular examination for documentation in the history sheet of the patient :

1. Examination for the head posture.
2. Examination of the forehead and face.
3. Examination of the eyebrows.
4. Examination of the eyelids.
5. Examination of the lacrimal apparatus.
6. Examination of the eyeballs as a whole to note any deviation, protrusion, size and movements of the eyeball.
7. Examination of all the parts of conjunctiva viz bulbar, palpebral and fornices.
8. Examination of cornea and fornices.
9. Examination of anterior chamber, iris and pupil.
10. Examination of the lens.
11. Measurement of intraocular pressure (tonometry).

III. FUNDUS EXAMINATION

This is performed to diagnose the diseases of the vitreous, optic nerve head, retina and choroid. For thorough examination of the fundus, pupils are to be fully dilated with 5 percent phenylepherine and/or 1 percent tropicamide eye drops. The fundus examination can be accomplished by ophthalmoscopy and focal illumination using a slit-lamp.

TECHNIQUES OF OCULAR EXAMINATION AND DIAGNOSTIC TESTS

LOUPE AND LENS EXAMINATION

It is a handy technique for examination of the anterior segment of the eye. It is performed in a semi-dark room using either a monocular corneal loupe (Fig. 2.4) or a binocular loupe (Fig. 2.5) and condensing lens of plus thirteen dioptre spherical. Fig.2.6 depicts the procedure of loupe and lens examination.

SLIT-LAMP EXAMINATION

Slit-lamp biomicroscopy forms an important part of ophthalmological examination. It allows minute examination of the various structures of the eyeball. A slit-lamp (Fig. 2.7) consists of following three parts :

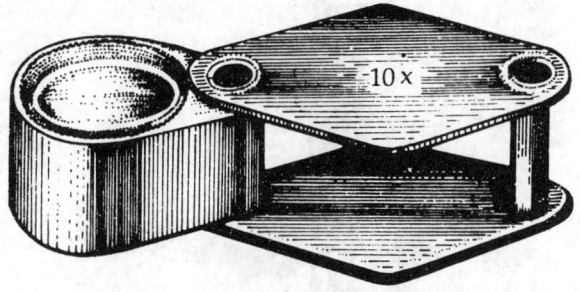

Fig. 2.4. Corneal loupe.

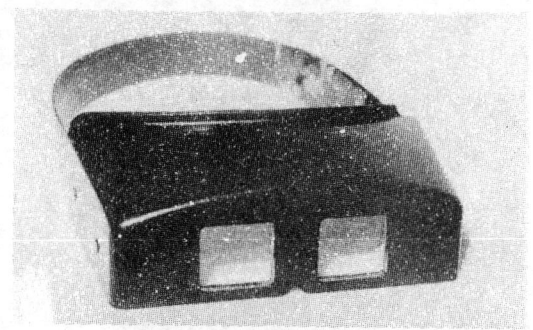

Fig. 2.5. Binocular loupe.

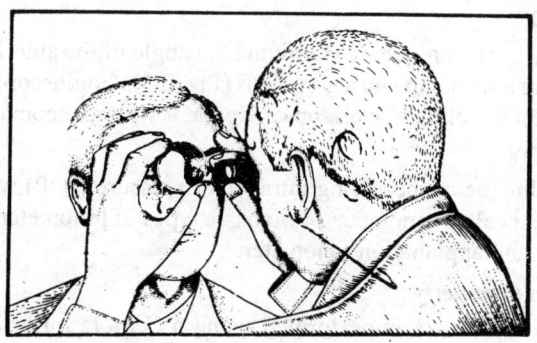

Fig. 2.6. Technique of loupe and lens examination.

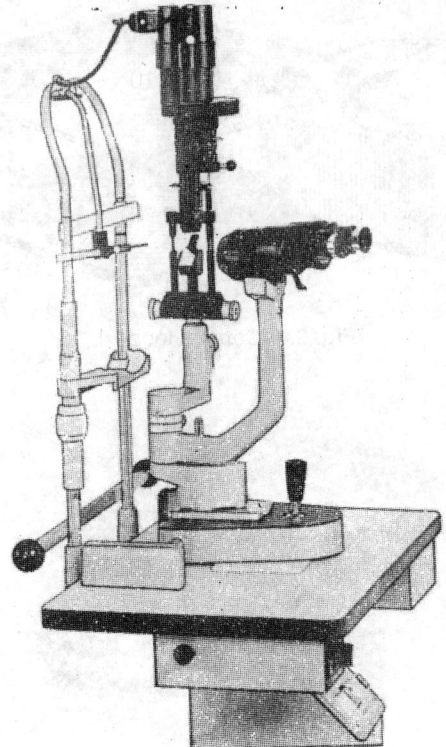

Fig. 2.7. A slit-lamp.

1. Observation system (microscope)
2. Illumination system (Slit-lamp)
3. Engineering support

GONIOSCOPY

Gonioscopy is a technique of examining the angle of the anterior chamber of eyeball using a slit-lamp and a goniolens (Fig. 2.8). Gonioscopic examination is essential in the clinical work up of a patient with glaucoma.

TONOMETRY

It is the technique of measuring intraocular pressure (IOP) with the help of an instrument called tonometer. Two basic types of tonometers available are indentation and applanation tonometer.

Indentation tonometry

Indentation tonometry is performed using a *Schiotz tonometer* (Fig. 2.9) which consists of following parts :

1. *Handle,* for holding the instrument in vertical position on cornea.
2. *Footplate* which rests on the cornea.

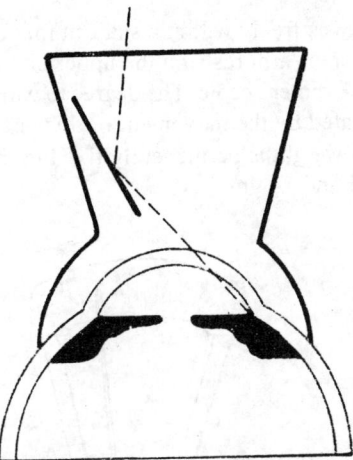

Fig. 2.8. Optics of gonioscopic examination with Goldmann's lens.

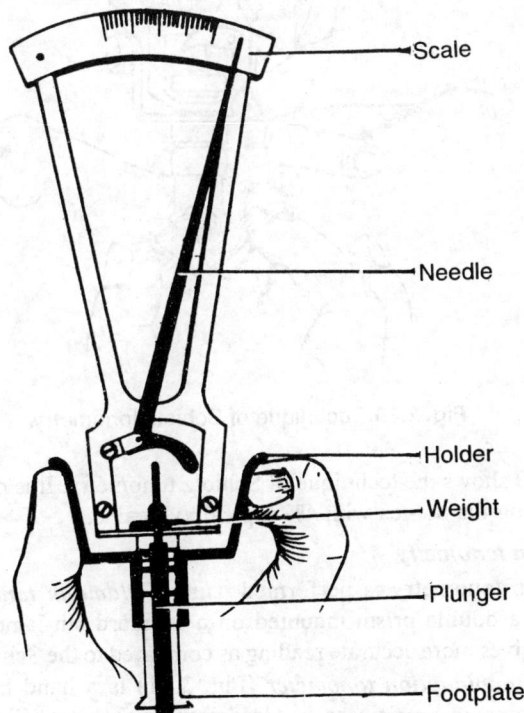

Fig. 2.9. Schiotz tonometer.

3. *Plunger,* which moves freely within a shaft in the footplate.
4. *Bent lever,* whose short arm rests on the upper end of plunger and a long arm which acts as a pointer needle. The degree to which the plunger indents the cornea is indicated by the movement of this needle on a scale.
5. *Weights.* A 5.5 gm weight is permanently fixed to the plunger, which can be increased to 7.5 and 10 gm.

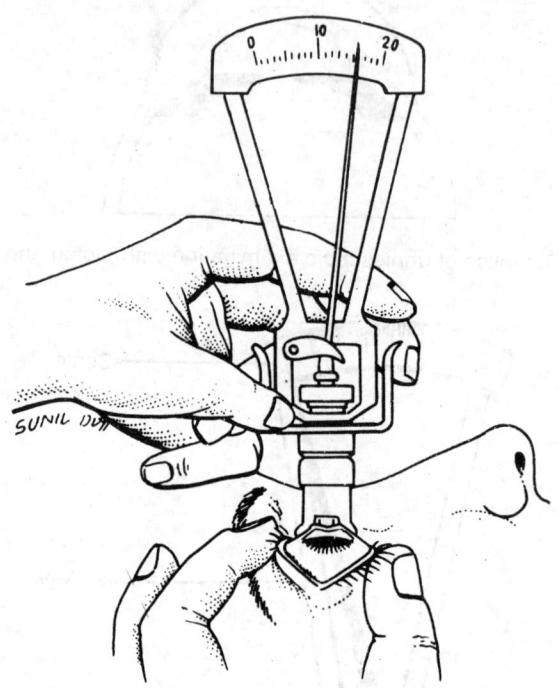

Fig. 2.10. Technique of Schiotz tonometry.

Fig. 2.10 shows the technique of Schiotz tonometry. It is performed after anaesthetising the cornea with 4% topical xylocaine.

Applanation tonometry

Applanation tonometry is performed using *Goldmann tonometer,* which consists of a double prism mounted on a standard slit-lamp. Applanation tonometer gives more accurate reading as compared to the Schiotz tonometer.

Perkin's applanation tonometer (Fig. 2.11) is a hand held tonometer utilizing the same biprism as in Goldmann tonometer. Fig 2.12 depicts technique of applanation tonometry.

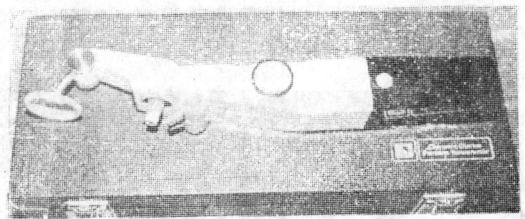

Fig. 2.11. Perkin's hand-held applanation tonometer

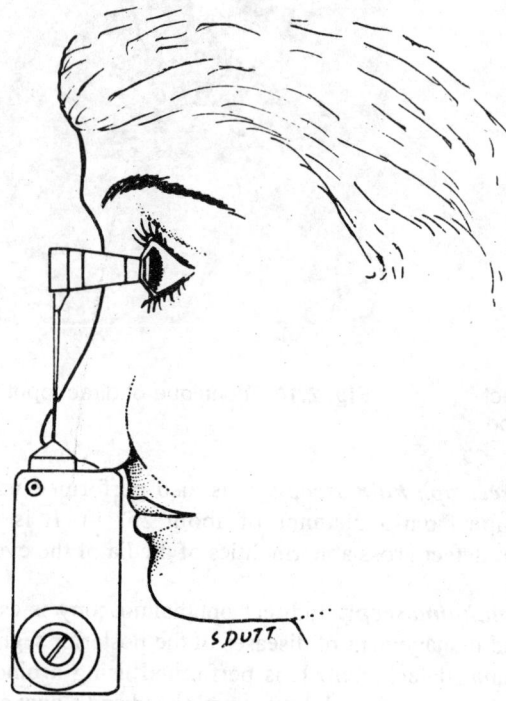

Fig. 2.12. Technique of applanation tonometry.

OPHTHALMOSCOPY

Ophthalmoscopy is the clinical examination of the interior of the eye (fundus) by means of an ophthalmoscope. It is of three types :

1. *Direct ophthalmoscopy*. It is the most commonly practised method for routine fundus examination using a direct ophthalmoscope (Fig. 2.13). Direct ophthalmoscopy is performed in a semidark room from a distance as close to the patient's eye as possible (Fig. 2.14)

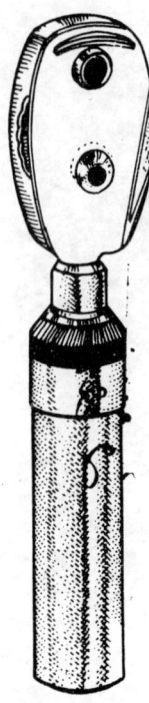

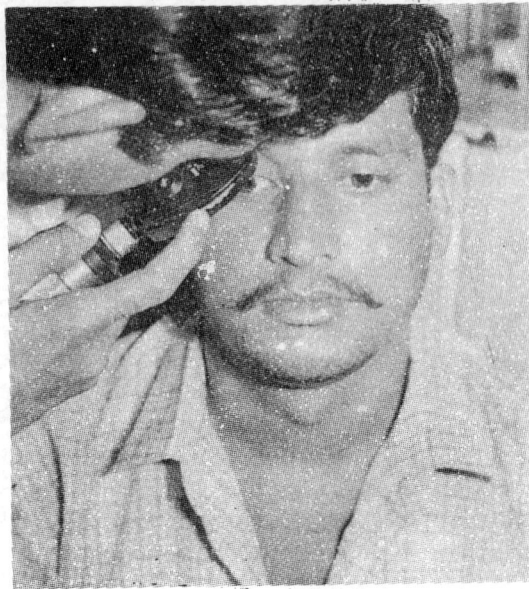

Fig. 2.13. Direct opthalmoscope

Fig. 2.14. Technique of direct ophthalmoscopy.

2. *Distant direct ophthalmoscopy.* It is also performed using the direct ophthalmoscope from a distance of about 25 cm. It is a preliminary examination to detect gross abnormalities of media of the eye.

3. *Indirect ophthalmoscopy.* Indirect ophthalmoscopy is essential for the assessment and management of diseases of the posterior segment of the eye especially retinal detachment. It is performed using a binocular indirect ophthalmoscope mounted on the examiner's head and a convex lens which is placed near the patient's eye (Fig.2.15)

PERIMETRY

Perimetry is the procedure of estimating extent of visual fields. The extent of normal visual field is superiorly –60°, inferiorly –70°, nasally –60° and temporally –90° (Fig. 2.16).

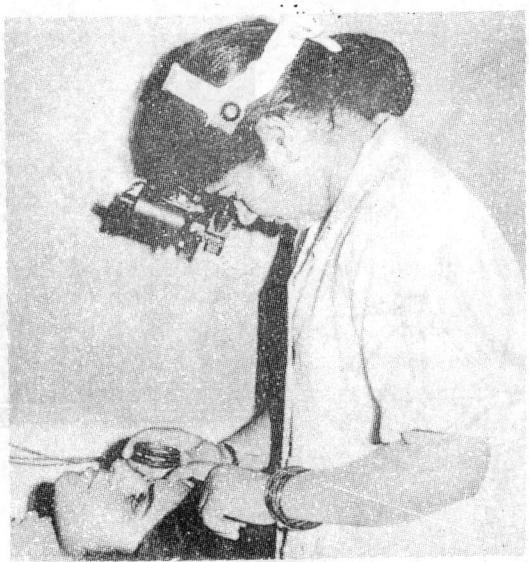

Fig. 2.15. Technique of indirect ophthalmoscopy.

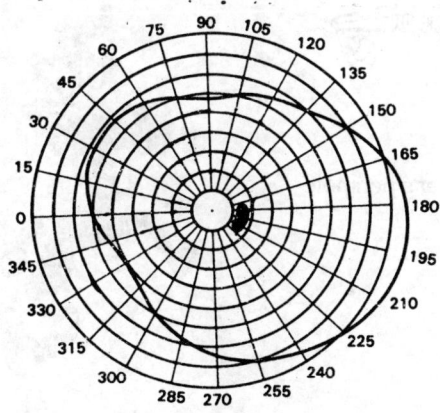

Fig. 2.16. Extent of normal visual field.

A few common methods of perimetry are as follows :

1. *Lister's perimeter* (Fig. 2.17). It is a simple and old perimeter used to measure the extent of peripheral fields. It has a metallic semicircular arc, graded in degrees, with a white dot for fixation in the centre. The arc can be rotated in different meridians.

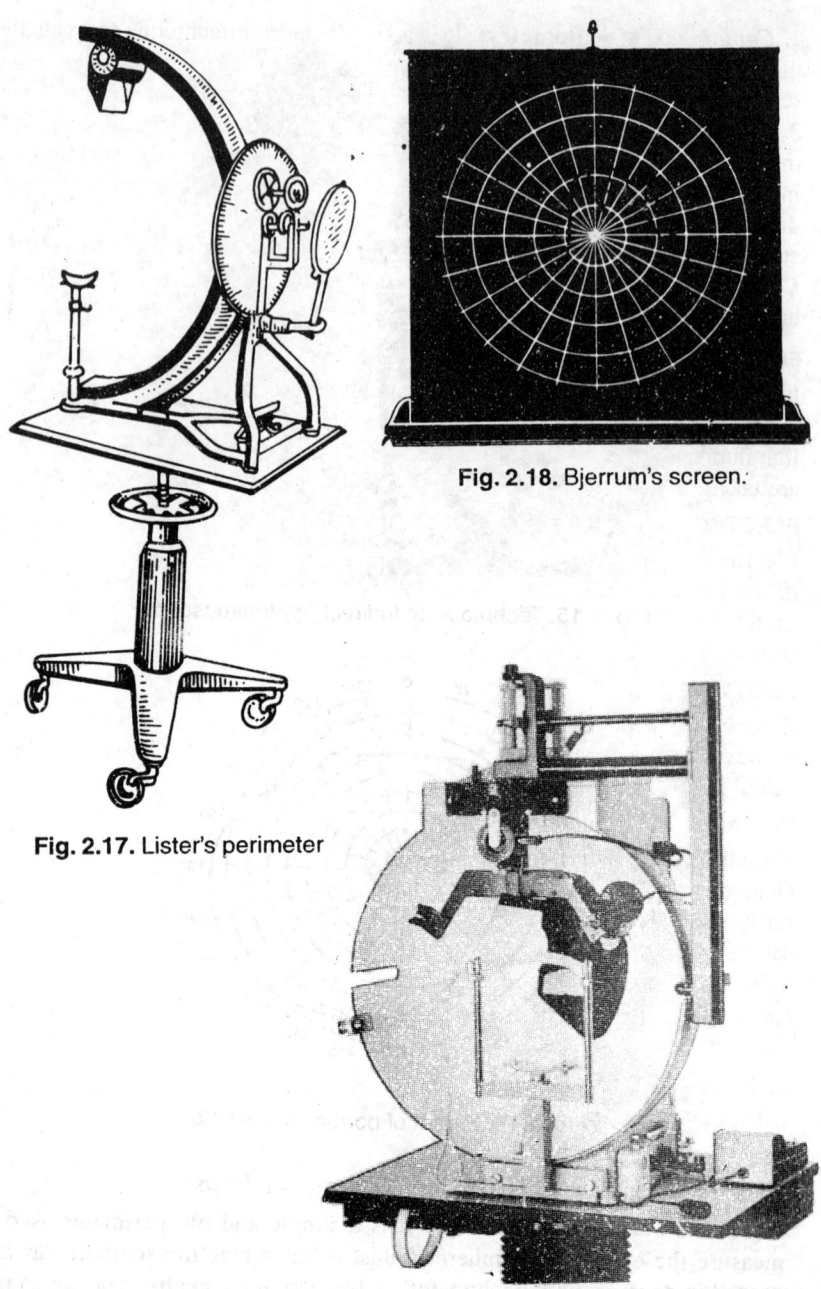

Fig. 2.18. Bjerrum's screen.

Fig. 2.17. Lister's perimeter

Fig. 2.19. Goldmann's perimeter.

2. Campimetry (Scotometry). It is a simple and old technique to evaluate the central and paracentral areas (30°) of the visual fields using the Bjerrum's screen (Fig. 2.18).

3. Goldmann perimeter (Fig. 2.19). It consists of a hemispherical dome. Its main advantage over the tangent screen is that the test conditions and the intensity of the target are always the same. It permits greater reproducibility.

4. Automated perimeters. There are computer assisted and automatically test suprathreshold and threshold stimuli and quantity depth of field defect. Commonly used automated perimeters are Octopus and Humphrey field analyser.

FUNDUS FLUORESCEIN ANGIOGRAPHY

It is a technique to study the various fundus disorders by observing changes in the flow of fluorescein dye along the vasculature of the retina and choroid. In it fluorescein dye is injected in the antecubical vein and serial photographs are taken on the fundus fluorescein angiography machine.

ELECTRORETINOGRAPHY

Electroretinography (ERG) is the record of changes in the resting potential of the eye induced by a flash light using an ERG machine. ERG is very useful in detecting the functional abnormalities of the outer retina, e.g. as seen in retinitis pigmentosa.

ELECTRO-OCULOGRAPHY

Electro-oculography (EOG) is based on the measurement of resting potential of the eye which exists between the cornea and back of the eye. It is also very useful in detecting the functional abnormalities of the outer retina.

VISUALLY EVOKED RESPONSE

Visually evoked response (VER) refers to the electroencephalographic (EEG) changes recorded at the occipital lobe. It is very useful in assessing the functional state of the visual pathway beyond the retinal ganglion cells. VER can be recorded by two techniques the **flash VER** and the pattern reversal VER.

OCULAR ULTRASONOGRAPHY

Ultrasonography has become a very useful diagnostic tool in ophthalmology. Both A and B scans are used. Common uses are :
1. Biometric study using A-scan to calculate power of intraocular lens (IOL) to be implanted.
2. Assessment of the posterior segment of the eyeball in the presence of opaque media.
3. Study of intraocular and orbital tumours.

NURSING PROCEDURES AND TECHNIQUES

A nurse may have to performe or assist some procedures performed in the ophthalmic out-patient clinics, indoors and operation theatre. A nurse must ensure that before carrying out any procedure, however simple, an explaination is given to the patient and he is made as comfortable as possible so that he is relaxed and able to cooperate. Some procedures are uncomfortable for the patient and others may be rather painful, but if the nurse has been able to gain his/her confidence various problems can generally be overcome. The common procedures are as follows :

SWABBING THE EYES

Swabbing of the eyes is a simple and the most common procedure to be performed by a nurse. It is required for cleaning the lid margin and stain of the lids of discharge, deposits of eye drops and eye ointments. To perform swabbing, a nurse should wash and dry her hands and then stand either behind or immediately in front of the seated patient, which ever is most convenient. Each eye should be swabbed with the eyelid gently closed by the patient first with swabs moistened in the normal saline solution and then, when the eyelids are thoroughly cleansed, with a dry swab. The eyelids should be swabbed from the outer canthus inwards and each swab used once only and then discarded.

INSTILLATION OF EYE DROPS AND OINTMENTS

Eye drops and ointments are of different types and instilled for various purposes; for example, to dilate the pupils (mydriatics), to constrict the pupils (miotics), to treat infections (antibiotics), to control inflammation (steroids and non-steroidal anti-inflammatory drugs) and so on. Therefore, before instilling the drugs, a nurse must ensure that she has the *correct patient,* the *correct medication* and the *correct eye.* Then she should tell the patient what she is going to do and how he should co-operate.

Technique. Position the patient in a horizontal supine position or have the patient sit with his neck hyperextended, looking towards the ceiling.

With the thumb or finger, pull down firmly on the lower eyelid with your left hand, having the patient look upward. This relaxes the upper tarsal plate or it is retracted into the orbit and exposes the lower conjunctival sac. Place one drop of medication into the lower conjunctival sac with your right hand (Fig. 2.20). Permit the patient to close his eye gently but not to squeeze. Wipe away excess tearing with a cotton ball or tissue. If more than one drop is to be instilled, permit the patient to close his eye between drops to permit the medication to be absorbed. In a crying infant, a drop may be placed in the inner canthus and then lower lid pulled down so that the drop rolls into the conjunctival sac.

If an eye ointment is to be used, express a ribbon of ointment long enough to cover the length of fornix from inner canthus to the outer canthus (Fig. 2.21). At the outer canthus, twist off the the ribbon by turning the tube. Ask the patient to gently clear the eyes. Spreading ointment along the lid margin is an effective way of getting ointment into a crying infant's eye.

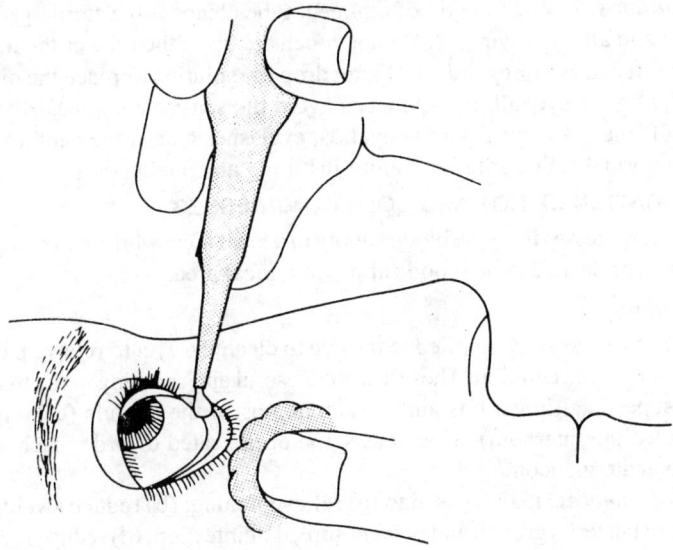

Fig. 2.20. Instillation of eye drops.

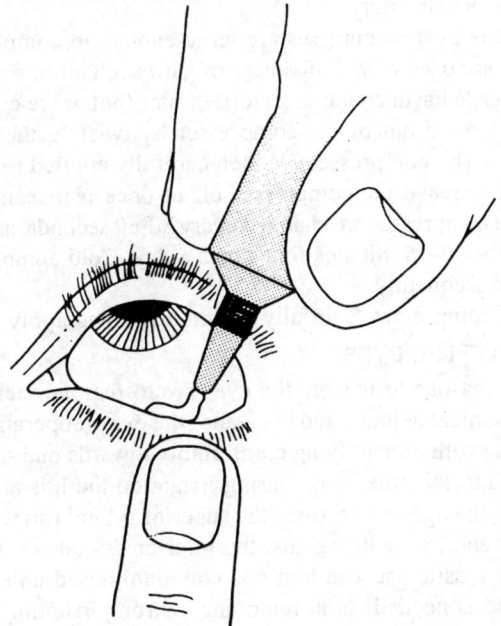

Fig. 2.21. Instillation of eye ointment.

Precautions. 1. Wipe the tip of ointment tube clean with a sterile gauze pad before and after applying. 2. Do not touch the tip of the tube or the tip of the dropper to the eye or eyelid. 3. Do not drop the solution or place the ointment directly on the eyeball. By all means avoid the sensitive cornea. 4. Always wipe off the ointment from the eyelids, eyelashes and in the canthus with a sterile normal saline solution before instilling any medication.

APPLICATION OF HOT AND COLD COMPRESSES

Warm compresses increase blood supply to a local area, while cold compresses constrict or decrease the blood supply to a local area.

Indications

1. *Hot compresses* are applied to the eye to clean the eye, to relieve pain, and to increase circulation. These are quite useful and soothing in the treatment of superficial infections and inflammations of the eyelids (e.g. stye and hordeolum internum), as well as some deep seated disorder such as iritis and acute glaucoma.
2. *Cold compress* may be used to (a) relieve itching; (b) reduce swelling; (c) retard bacterial growth and prevent spread of infection; (d) reduce secretion; (e) relieve pain; (f) prevent or control oedema; and (g) help control bleeding.
   Cold compresses are useful in inflammatory and allergic conjunctivitis and following ocular injuries.

Technique. The best compresses are large enough to completely cover the eye and are composed of 7-8 thickness of gauze or cotton flannel. These are dipped in a sterile basin containing sterile water (hot or ice cold). The excess solution is removed out of the compresser by twisting them between two sterile forceps. The compresses are then carefully applied to the closed eye. Care is taken to leave the compresser off at once if it feels too hot to the patient. Warm compresses are changed every 30-60 seconds, and the treatment is continued for 10-15 minutes four times a day. Cold compresses need not be changed so frequently.

Following compresses, carefully dry the eyes, and apply medication.

IRRIGATION OF THE EYES

The common reasons to irrigate the eyes are to remove secretions, foreign bodies and chemical irritants and to cleanse the eye preoperatively. Irrigation should be done with patient lying comfortably towards one side so that fluid can not flow into the other eye. During irrigation the lids are kept open by firmly holding the upper lid against the superior orbital rim with the index or middle finger and lower lid against the inferior orbital rim with the thumb (Fig. 2.22). A plastic squeeze bottle is commonly used unless a very large amount is fluid is needed, as in removing a strong irritating chemical from the eye. Under such conditions a bigger container or even a direct top water may be used to irrigate the eyes. The aim is not to dilute but remove the whole caustic material by copiously washing the eye.

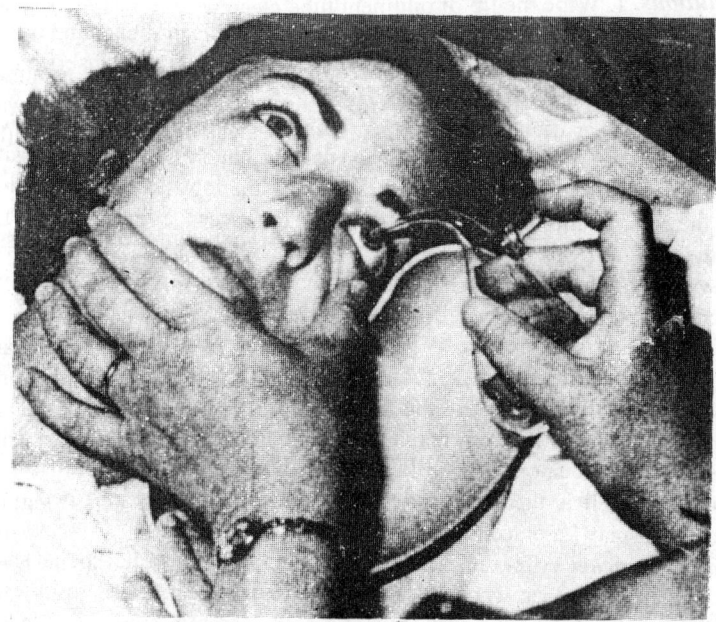

Fig. 2.22. Irrigation of the eye using an undine.

Physiologic solution of sodium chloride or lactated Ringer's solution is most often used as irrigating solution. These solution are isotonic and do not remove from the eye secretions the electrolytes necessary for normal health of the eyes. For preoperative irrigation of the eye, 1 in 10 dilutions of betadine solution filled in a 10 or 20 ml syringe is preferred.

Irrigating fluid should be directed along the conjunctiva and over the eyeball from the inner to the outer canthus. Care should be taken to avoid directing a forceps stream on to the eyeball and to avoid touching any eye structures with the irrigating equipment.

INSERTION, REMOVAL AND CARE OF AN ARTIFICIAL EYE

An artificial eye or the ophthalmic prosthesis is used for cosmetic purposes in patients where eyeball has been enucleated, eviscerated or has shrunken. (phthisis bulbi) because of disease process.

To begin with, staff nurse has to insert, remove and care for the socket and artificial eye of the patient. She has also to teach the patient or parent (in case of a child) the whole procedure. Since the prosthesis is a foreign object, it must be removed and cleaned daily. If it is neglected, slight discharge can occur.

Insertion of the prosthesis. The artifical eye should be worked thoroughly and inserted wet to reduce friction between the prosthesis and conjunctiva lining the orbit. Because it is imporant to maintain a clean socket and prevent infection, it is essential that one's hands be washed before insertion and removal of the eye.

To insert the artificial eye the upper lid is lifted and pulled slightly upward and the upper portion of the prosthesis is slipped under it as far as possible. Then, supporting the prosthesis with left hand, the lower lid is pulled down with the right thumb or index finger until it slips over the lower edge of the prosthesis.

Removal of the prosthesis. It is important that removable artificial eye should be removed at night before retiring and cleansed thoroughly.

The prosthesis is removed by gently depressing the lower lid and exerting a small amount of pressure under the lower edge of the prosthesis. The prosthesis will then slip out of the orbit because the suction is broken.

Care of the prosthesis. Immediately after the prosthesis is removed, it is placed in a sterile sponge basin lined with gauze pads and is cleansed with normal saline. It is then stored in a safe place on a clean soft bed of dry cotton, or it may be placed in a solution of normal saline.

Care of the socket. After removal of the artificial eye the orbital socket should be irrigated with clean water and soaked dry with clean towel followed by instillation of 2-3 drops of antibiotic eye drops. To minimize the formation of secretions in the socket, the prosthesis should be lubricated with commercially available ophthalmic solutions.

NURSING CARE OF AN EYE PATIENT

GENERAL GUIDELINES FOR NURSING CARE OF OPHTHALMIC PATIENTS

1. Before undertaking any treatment the nurse should explain what she is about to do to the patient in order to gain his confidence and cooperation.
2. When approaching a patient who is unable to see, the nurse should speak quitely to him by name in order to make her presence known, and when walking with him should allow him to hold her lightly by the arm if he is unfamiliar with the surroundings.
3. The nurse should play a key role in teaching the patient and attendants about general eye care and protection of vision.
4. The ophthalmic nurse must be gentle and dextrous in using her hands when carrying out procedures.
5. Always wash hands before and after performing procedures related to the eyes.
6. Maintain aseptic technique to protect an unaffected eye from cross-infection.
7. Do not exert pressure over the eyeball when performing ocular procedures.

8. Always open the eyelids by pressing against the bony orbit rather than directly against the eyeball.
9. Provide appropriate safety measures for the blind or partially sighted (including patients with binocular bandage). For example, when the patient is in bed, keep side rails up.
10. Instruct patients to never touch their eyes, eye dressing or eye shields. Rubbing the eyes may cause injury or introduce infection.
11. An ophthalmic staff nurse should familiarize her self with general guidelines concerning ocular medicatioins and with specific eye medications.
12. The ophthalmic nurse should be familiar with basic ocular disorder, their symptoms and common treatments both medical as well as surgical (these have been described in the ensuing chapters).

NURSING CARE OF THE NON-SEEING PATIENT

1. The first step in care for the nonseeing patient is to tell him your name and that you are a nurse. State your purpose for coming. Address the non-seeing patient by name so that he will know that you are talking to him. Do not touch a nonseeing patient before announcing your presence as this will surely startle him. This should also be conveyed to the family, as their first impulse is to reach out and touch the loved one. Remember that the patient does not know who is walking around his bed. Are you someone who can give him a glass of water or a relaxing backrub? Will you relieve his monotonous day with a cheerful word? Can you be an intruder seeking his wallet? Are you a window washer passing through his room to invade his privacy while he is bathing?

2. Whatever is done will require somewhat more explanation than that required for a seeing patient. Specific instructions may also be needed in defining how the patient may assist in his own care, and repeated instructions may be needed throughout the day, depending upon the nursing activity involved. Speak directly and clearly to the patient, but do not shout; his sensory deprivation is sight, not hearing. Effective use of both verbal and nonverbal communication does much to convey understanding. A nod of your head, a smile, or a wink are not enough - a patient must be given words, he must be given expression and feeling. He cannot see the sincere concern reflected in your eyes, but he can hear it in your voice and feel it in your touch. Your physical contact with the patient and physical proximity when talking to him suggests your interest in him. Conversation should be natural without consciously avoiding words such as "see" and "eyes". When you leave the patient, let him know that you are going as well as if and when you will return. Both seeing and nonseeing individuals find it embarrassing to talk into thin air.

3. It is important to remember that the paitent may find himself totally dependent on less used senses such as hearing and touch. It is through these senses that orientation to surroundings will be achieved. If, for instance, the patient is to bathe himself, all necessary items must be placed within arm's around him. Do not hurry the patient. Tell him precisely where and how far away he will find the washbowl, chair, door, or obstacles. Most people make the mistake of trying to push a blind patient. It is bad enough to be blind, without being pushed around also ! Place the blind person's hand upon your elbow. In this way it is possible to guide him inconspicuously simply by walking at a normal pace and being certain no obstacles to head or foot threaten the patient's safety. Stairways should be announced in advance.

5. Do not leave a blind patient in a strange room without orienting him to the surroundings. The bedfast patient with bandaged eyes should have the nurse's call button fastened to the sheet near his hand. The call button should always be placed in the same location so that if the patient needs it quickly, he will not have to search for it. Knowledge of handedness will be a determining factor in its placement. If the patient cannot use an electric call button, a small bell can be substituted. Reminding the patient that he can always loudly call out for help is reassuring. The patient who may care for himself should be guided to the sink and to the bathroom and should have his hand placed on the soap, paper towels, toilet paper, etc.

6. Perhaps as important as anything else, especially in the area of safety, is that the blind person must never be permitted to smoke unattended in bed. Although the nurse may be tempted to leave when a patient has half finished a cigarette without difficulty, she should remember that he would almost certainly sustain serious burns in the event of a fire. Many patients find it easier to use the metal emesis basin as an ashtray because of the depth and size rather than the small glass ashtrays found in most hospitals.

7. Patients who are bilaterally patched usually feel more secure when both side rails are up. If it is necessary to leave a patient with one of the side rails down, let the patient know. For patients who are unilaterally patched the side rails are usually left down, provided their condition permits. Objects of personal use are placed within reach on the bedside table.

8. Mealtime should be an anticipated time of diversion for the nonseeing patient, but it can also prove to be a real problem. Lack of activity, lack of independence in being able to feed himself and lack of visual stimulation by food may all contribute to a decreased appetite. The meal tray should be described – the position of the utensils, the milk, and the various items of food. The patient should be asked what food he would like to start with, as we have varied eating patterns. Encouraging the patient to help himself, such as with bread, bacon, and other finger foods, helps to promote a feeling of independence. Thin cereals and soups can be sipped through

a straw or drunk from a cup. Hot foods should be served hot and cold foods cold since it is most disconcerting to eat a lukewarm meal. Mealtime provides the nurse with an opportunity to discuss normal nutrition or modified diets that the patient may be receiving. For patients who are temporarily patched the most significant factor relative to nutrition is hydration. Even if the patient does not eat during the period of bed confinement, this is usually so short that no serious nutritional problems will develop. However, it is imperative that the fluid intake be adequate. If necessary, liquids high in nutritional value can be provided frequently throughout the day.

9. When giving a medication to the patient, tell him in advance if it is a pill or a liquid. If you are administering an injection, tell the patient and let him know what he can do to assist. He cannot see what you have on your medicine tray, and the shock of receiving an injection without being forewarned can be unnerving.

10. Finding a pleasant way of passing the time is frequently a problem for the nonseeing patient. He cannot read or watch television and may not even be aware that other patients are around with whom he can talk. This is an area in which you can sincerely show your interest, even as you go about your daily activities. A cheerful "hello" as you pass through his room, and stopping at his bedside for a few moments to talk will relieve the dull, heavy hours. A radio at the bedside is an appropriate and often a helpful diversion.

PREOPERATIVE NURSING CARE

Preoperative nursing care and treatment varies with the hospital, the eye surgeon, the operation to be performed, age of the patient (child or an adult) and the personality of an adult patient. Some guidelines for preoperative nursing care are as follows :

1. *Information and consent about operation.* An explaination of the surgery to be performed is always given by the eye surgeon. However, if the patient has any further questions, the nurse should clarify these only after ascertaining what the physician has already told the patient or parents of the child about the operation and the reason for it and the risks involved in it. A written consent about detailed information should be taken.

If the surgery requires a *local anaesthesia* the patient should be told that he will be awake during the procedure but will feel no pain and that he should hold his head still during surgery.

In case surgery is to be performed under general anaesthesia, patient should be advised to omit food and fluid by mouth since the preceding night.

2. *Orient and familiarize the patient* with the surroundings, other staff and patients, especially if the patient is going to have binocular bandage or bandage on the only eye. Familiarizing the patient with his surroundings preoperatively not only makes the patient generally more comfortable psychologically but also may specifically lessen postoperative disorientation. This appears particularly true of elderly people.

3. *Preoperative preparation and medications.* The eye to be operated should be marked properly as per the routine of institution and if ordered eyelashes should be cut. A nurse should give the eye drops and other medications as per orders *at the precise time.* The specific medication order vary depending upon the type of surgery and type of anaesthesia to be given.

4. *Preoperative general care instructions* include to take cleaning both, to shave (for male patients) and to comb and braid the hair if it is long. Before being taken to the operating room, precaution such as the removal of jewellary and dentures, houring the patient void, etc., must be taken.

POSTOPERATIVE NURSING CARE

Like preoperative nursing cases, considerable variations exist concerning post-operative nursing care as well depending upon the hospital, the surgeon, type of surgery and the type of anaesthesia. In general, many recent advances in ocular surgery have revolutionized the postoperative nursing care. The major goals of nursing care following intraocular surgery are to (a) prevent hemorrhage; (b) prevent stress on the suture line; (c) prevent increased intraocular pressure; (d) prevent infection, and (e) prevent complications of immobility and anaesthesia. Some guidelines for post operative nursing care as below :

1. *Immediate postoperative nursing care when operation is performed under general anaesthesia* include :
- Care of the vitals – pulse, respiration and blood pressure.
- Maintenance of intravenous fluids.
- Nil orally for six hours.
- Injectable analgesics and anti-emetics for postoperative pain and vomiting.
- Care should be taken that the dressing is not loosened or removed.

2. *Immediate postoperative nursing care* when operation has been performed under local anaesthesia includes :
- The patient must keep the head still and try to avoid coughing, vomiting snezing or moving suddenly.
- The patient should lie with the unoperated side down to prevent pressure on the operated eye and to prevent possible contamination of the dressing with vomitus, in case vomiting occurs.
- Vitals – respiration, pulse and blood pressure must be checked after the operation.
- Nil orally for about ½–1 hours.
- To prevent postoperative pain, which usually starts after 1 hour operation, oral analgesic may be given.

3. *Bedrest and ambulation.* Years ago it was necessary for a patient to lie flat in bed for ten days with his head immobilized by sand bags after cataract surgery. With the development of better microsurgical techniques and finer suture material and recently even sutureless surgery under topical anaesthesia (phacoemulsification) it is now possible for the patient to be up and around one hour after the surgery. Infact the cataract operation has become now a day-care surgery. With early ambulation the complications associated with recumbent position in elderly have been reduced markedly.

Bed rest in specific position may be ordered in some complicated cases of retinal detachment surgery. If a patient has to remain on prolonged bed rest for one or the other reason , it is important for the nurse to ensure that the patient continues frequently to perform isometric exercises and that other appropriate care is administered to prevent the complications of prolonged inactivity. Frequent deep breathing sessions to clear lens and frequent position changes are also important.

4. *Routine activities* are now-a-days allowed very early following ocular surgery. However, activities which increase intraocular pressure are contraindicated after intraocular surgery. These include excessive energy exertion, crying, extreme emotion, sudden movements, sneezing, coughing, running, jumping, lifting or pushing heavy objects, rubbing the eyes and lightly closing the eyes.

The nurse caring for the patient in the hospital has a responsibility to teach the patient how to follow these instructions when the patient is most receptive to teaching.

5. *Diet and feeding.* Patients who received a local anaesthetic are permitted a soft diet within an hour of operation. Those who received a general anaesthesia are first placed on intravenous fluids, then on a liquid diet postnauses, progressing gradually to a regular diet.

Diet must be light until the bowels are open and after this heavy rich foods are undesirable. Soups, meat essences, eggs, milk, custards, jelly, thin bread and butter, milk puddings, soft fruits, fruit juices and tea etc. are example of suitable food articles in the immediate few postoperative days.

When patients are accustomed to alcohol their usual beverage must be continued in a quantity below their normal intake, but no drastic reduction should be made for heavy drinkers on account of risk of delirium tremens.

Patients with bilateral banadage or otherwise not able to eat themselves should be fed by a nurse with great affection. The nurse who undertakes the feeding must exercise great patience and make arrangements to keep hot food warm during this slow process.

6. *Postoperative medications* should be used by the nurse as per the orders by the ophthalmologist. A nurse should observe sterile techniques while instilling eye drops and ointments and for all procedures performed on the eye following intraocular surgery. The development of intraocular infection is a serious complication.

7. *Instructions at discharge and homegoing preparation.* Instruction for home-going regimen are prescribed by the surgeon. However, the nurse has a responsibility to ascertain the patient's understanding of the physician's orders. Prior to discharge, she should make emphasis on following points :

- The patient (and family) should be made to understand the *restrictions* which are necessary to prevent elevation of intraocular pressure and see that he is familiar with *home care procedures* e.g., instillation of eye drops.
- Sponge bath may be necessary for a period of time at home.
- It may be desirable for the patient to wear metal eye sheild or eye-pad at night or when lying down resting to protect his eye.
- Dark glasses may work for a while following removal of eye dressings to protect the eyes from bright sunlight.
- Instruct that patient who will be wearing any type of glasses postoperatively that he should hold his glasses by the tips of their bows when putting them on to avoid accidentally poking his eye.
- Teach the patient how to properly care for eye glasses and/or contact lenses.
- Instruct the patient to grasp both arms of a chain before sitting down to prevent slipping and possibility of falling.
- Emphasize to the patient that he should not rub his eyes with a soiled handkerchief.
- Be certain the patient realizes the importance of keeping follow-up appointments with his physician and the necessity of contacting the doctor whenever untoward symptoms develop.
- If enucleation has been performed, the patient must be instructed regarding the use and care of an artificial eye.

ROLE OF A NURSE IN OPHTHALMIC OPERATION THEATRE

1. *Preoperative nursing care* which stands in the ophthalmic word continues in the pre-medication room of the operation theatre as well. A nurse should be familiar with the measures already described and also about the specific medication/preparation required for different operative procedures to be performed.

2. *Handling and care of instruments.* A nurse should be familiar with laying down of the instrument trolley, care of instruments and general principles of sterility to be maintained in the operation theatre. She also needs to be familiar with the various instruments and the operative steps of different ocular operations where the particular instrument is required. Commonly used ophthalmic instruments are described on page 52.

3. *Immediate postoperative nursing care* as discussed earlier, is to be carried out by the staff nurse posted in operation theatre.

ROLE OF A NURSE IN MOBILE EYE CLINIC AND EYE CAMPS

Eye camp approach for prevention of blindness still plays a vital role in the developing countries where infrastructure is not fully established. A nurse has to play a pivotal role in eye camps. She may be required to carry out any of the following duties :

1. To assist the eye surgeon in examination of the patients.
2. To deliver instructions on eye health care and ocular hygiene.
3. To carry out preoperative and postoperative nursing care of the patients admitted for operations.
4. To assist the eye surgeons in operating rooms.
5. To handle and care the instruments used for eye surgery.

Basic Principles of Ocular Therapy

A staff nurse has to play a very important role in the management of patients; so she needs to be familiar with the various modalities employed in the management of patients suffering from eye diseases. These modalities are :

- Pharmacotherapy (Medical management),
- Ocular surgery
- Laser therapy, and
- Cryotherapy

Modern ophthalmology has reached a stage, where medical, surgical, laser and cryotherapy are playing an almost equal role in the management of eye diseases. Basic principles of those modalities are discussed.

OCULAR PHARMACOTHERAPY

The nurse working in an ophthalmic unit should be familiar with the action of commonly used eye drops and ointments. She must also be able to instruct patients clearly and concisely how to use these at home.

OPHTHALMIC MEDICATIONS

The agents commonly used in ophthalmology include :

- Antimicrobial agents
- Antibiotics
- Antiviral drugs
- Antifungal drugs
  - Anti-glaucoma drugs
  - Corticosteroids
  - Non-steroidal anti-inflammatory drugs
  - Local anaesthetics
  - Viscoelastic substances
  - Diagnostic stains
  - Miscellaneous

ANTIMICROBIAL AGENTS

Antimicrobial agents for use in eye are normally applied topically as eye drops or eye ointments; but occasionally sub-conjunctival and intravitreal injections are used. Antibiotics are also used systemically in certain eye diseases.

Antibiotics

Commonly available antibiotic eye drops and ointments (along with their strength) are as follows :

- Ciprofloxacin (0.3% eye drops and eye ointment).
- Norfloxacin (0.3% eye drops and eye ointment).
- Gentamycin (0.3% eye drops and eye ointment).
- Neomycin sulfate (0.25 to 0.5% eye drops)
- Framycetine (0.5% eye drops and ointment)
- Tetracycline (1% eye ointment)
- Chloramphemicol (0.5% – 1% eye drops and 1% eye ointment)
- Neosporine eye drops and ointment (Combination of neomycin, polymyxin and bacitracin)
- Polymyxin B sulfate (0.25% eye drops or 0.21% ointment)
- Erythomycin (1% ointment)

Sulfonamides

- Sulfacetamide is used as 10, 20 or 30% eye drops for chlamydial infections especially trachoma.

Antiviral drugs

- *Idoxuridine* (0.1% eye drops or 0.5% eye ointment) is effective against herpes simplex infections.
- *Acyclovir* (3% eye ointment) is effective against both herpes simplex and herpes zoster infection.

Anti fungal drugs

- Nystatin (3.5% eye ointment)
- Natamycin (5% eye drops)
- Fluconazole (% eye drops)
- Silver sulfadiazine (% eye drops)

Mydriatics and cycloplegics

Mydriatic drugs dilate the pupil and cycloplegics paralyse the ciliary muscles and prevent the process of accommodation.

Uses

- Short-term dilatation of the pupil for examination of the fundus and for operation of cataract.
- Long term treatment for keratitis, iritis or iridocyclitis.
- On occasion, after operative treatment or accidental trauma

Preparation

1. *Atropine* (1% eye drops or ointment).
   It is the strongest acting cycloplegic drug. The affect of atropine may last for more than a week.
2. *Homatropine* (2% eye drops). Its effect last for 24-48 hours.
3. *Cyclopentolate* (1% eye drops) It is a short acting cycloplegia. Its effect lasts for 6-18 hour.
4. *Tropicamide.* It is the shortest acting cycloplegic. It is a very good mydriatic drug and so is often used for short term dilation of pupils.

Antiglaucoma Drugs

These drugs lower the intraocular pressure. These include the following:

1. *Miotics*

Miotics are parasympathomimetic drugs. The most commonly used preparation is *Pilocarpine* (1,2,4% eye drops). It is useful in the treatment of primary open angle as well as primary narrow angle glaucoma. Other preparations are: *Carbachol* (0.75% and 3% eye drops), *Ecothiophate* (0.03, 0.00 and 0.125% eye drops) and *Physostigmine* (0.5% eye ointment).

2. *Sympathomimetic drugs*

Sympathomimetic or the adrenergic drugs which are used as antiglaucoma agents are :
− Epinephrine (0.5, 1.0 and 2% eye drops)
− Dipivefrine (0.1% eye drops)
− Apraclonidine (0.5% eye drops)
− Brimonidine (0.2% eye drops)

3. *Beta blockers*

These are presently the most frequently used antiglaucoma drugs preparations available are :
− Timolol (0.25 and 0.5% eye drops)
− Betoxalal (0.25 and 0.5% eye drops)
− Levobunolol (0.5% eye drops)

4. *Carbonic anhyrase inhibitors (CAI)*

− *Acetazolamide* (250 mg tablet)
− Dorzolamide (% eye drops)

5. *Hyperosmotic agents*

Glycerol It is used as 5% solution orally.
Mannitol. It is used as 20% solution intravenously.

Anti-inflammatory drugs

Corticosteroids

Corticosteroids have potent anti-inflammatory, anti-allergic and anti-fibrotic actions. These may be administered locally in the form of eye drops, eye ointments or subconjunctival injections and systemically in the form of tablets and injections.

Topical preparations

- Hydrocortisone acetate (0.5% suspension and 0.2% solution).
- Dexamethasone (0.1% eye drops and 0.5% ointment)
- Beta methasone (0.1% eye drops and 0.1% eye ointment)

Non-steroidal anti-inflammatory drugs

- Indomethacin suspension (0.1%)
- Flurbiprofen (0.3% eyedrops)
- Ketorolac tromethamine (0.5% eye drops)
- Diclofenac sodium (o.1% eye drops)

Viscoelastic substances

Viscoelastic substances are used in the modern intraocular microscopic surgery especially intraocular lens implantation.

Preparations

- Methycellulose (2%)
- Sodium hyaluronate (1%)
- Hypromellose (2%)

Local anaesthetics

Xylocaine (1,2 and 4%) is the most commonly employed local anaesthetic. In the eye it can be used as eye drops (2-4%) for topical anaesthesia and as injection (1-2%) for retrobulbar block, facial block and peribulbar block anaesthesia.

Diagnostic stains

Corneal damage, either from an ulcer or following trauma, is more readily assessed if a stain or dye is instilled into the eye before examination. These include :

– *Fluorescein dye.* It stains the disrupted epithelium as pale yellowish-green.
– *Bengal rose.* It stains the dead cells as pink.

GUIDELINES FOR USING OPHTHALMIC MEDICATION

1. Never instill medication into the eye unless it is ordered by a physician.
2. *Do not use "old" medications,* i.e. those that have been on the shelf for a long while. Check the expiry date on the medication. Two weeks is a reasonable time to use a solution before discarding it. Date the bottle at the time it is procured from pharmacy.
3. *Before using ocular solutions,* e.g. "eye drops," *inspect them,* e.g. for cloudiness, discoloration, and precipitation. If precipitate is present or if the solution is cloudy or discolored, do not use it.
4. *Follow package instructions concerning proper storage of eye medications.*

5. *Obtain new stock solutions weekly.* Medications most likely to become contaminated are fluorescein, tetracaine (Pentacaine), proparacaine (Ophthaine, Ophthetic), and physostigmine.

6. *Ophthalmic solutions must be sterile.* They are prepared and handled with the same degree of caution against contamination that is given to fluids intended for I.V. administration. Use sterile medications supplied in sterile, disposable, single-use eyedropper units if the eye has been injured (accidentally or surgically).

7. *Use eyedroppers correctly.* Do not use the same eyedropper to instill two different medications. Do not allow medication in an eye dropper to flow back into the dropper's bulb, and do not return medication remaining in the eyedropper back into the bottle after instillation. Such practices cause contamination of the medication.

8. *Check carefully which medication is to be instilled in which eye.* Different medications may be ordered for each of the two eyes.

9. *Familiarize yourself with specific eye medications.* Certain medications are definitely contraindicated for certain eye disorders.

10. *Never substitute a solution or medication of one strength for that of another strength without permissiion from the physician.* Also, never substitute one eye medication for another without permission.

11. *Carefully read instructions and labels for all ocular medications* (and any other ocular treatment). If labels are smeared or otherwise unreadable discard them or return them to pharmacy for relabeling.

12. *Never use an unlabeled solution or ointment on the eye or around the eye.*

OPHTHALMIC SURGERY

Eye surgery is now-a-days very much advanced and is a modality for successful management of many ocular diseases such as cataract, glaucoma, squint etc. A nurse should be familiar with the various ocular operations which have been described along with the diseases in the ensuring chapters. She has to play an important role in the pre-operative and postoperative nursing care of such patients which have been described on page 41 & 42 and, respectively. Role of a nurse in eye operation theatre has been discussed on page 44.

ESSENTIAL EQUIPMENT FOR OPHTHALMIC OPERATION THEATRE

In addition to the basic requirements of general operation theatre with equipment for general anaesthesia and facilities to deal with the cardio-respiratory emergency situations, a modern ophthalmic operation theatre should also have the following equipment: an operating microscope (Fig. 3.1), an ophthalmic cryo unit (Fig. 3.2), a wet-field bipolar cautery, an electrolysis machine, an electromagnetic unit for removal of intraocular foreign bodies, a vitrectomy unit and preferably a phacoemul sification machine for modern cataract surgery.

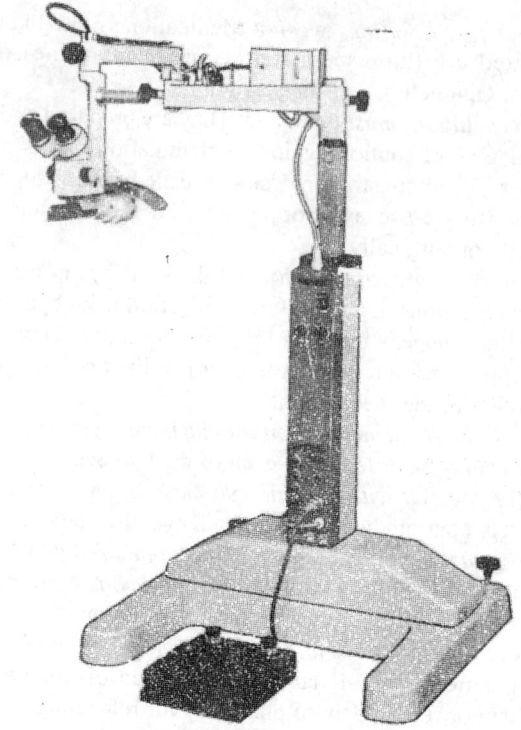

Fig. 3.1. Operating microscope.

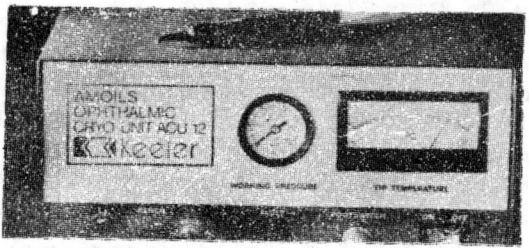

Fig. 3.2. Ophthalmic cryo unit.

OPHTHALMIC INSTRUMENTS

Commonly used ophthalmic instruments can be grouped as under:

I. Lid speculums

These are used to keep the lids apart during any operation on the eyeball.
Three types of speculums are in use:

1. *Universal eye speculum* (Fig. 3.3).

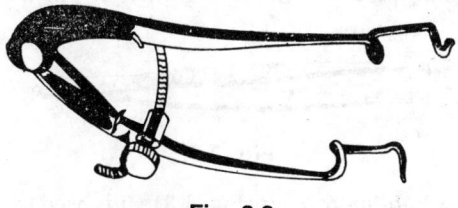

Fig. 3.3.

2. *Eye speculum with guard* (Fig. 3.4).

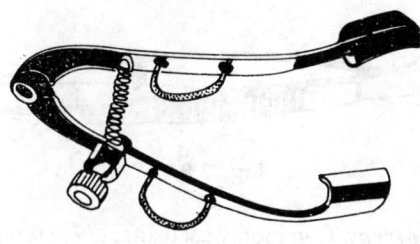

Fig. 3.4.

3. *Wire speculum* (Fig. 3.5).

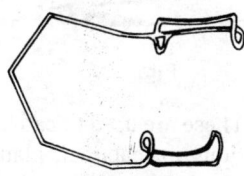

Fig. 3.5

II. Forceps

1. ***Plain forceps*** (Fig. 3.6). It is simple forceps without any teeth, *used* to hold the conjunctiva during any surgical procedure.

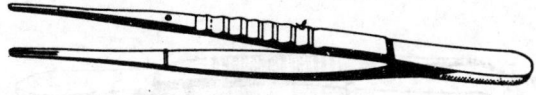

Fig. 3.6.

2. **Globe fixation forceps** (Fig. 3.7). It is applied near the limbus to hold the conjunctiva and episcleral tissue together, to fix the eyeball during operations.

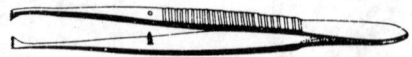

Fig. 3.7.

3. **Superior rectus holding forceps** (Fig. 3.8). It is used to hold the superior rectus muscle while passing a suture under it; to stabilize the eyeball during any operation such as cataract surgery, glaucoma surgery, corneal surgery etc.

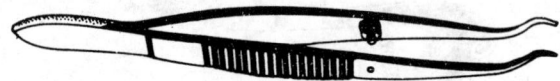

Fig. 3.8

4. **Corneo-scleral forceps.** Commonly used are *colibri forceps* (Fig. 3.9) and *Lim's forceps*. These are used to hold the corneal or scleral edge (of incision) for suturing during cataract, glaucoma and keratoplasty operations.

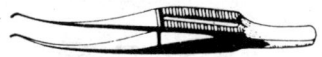

Fig. 3.9.

5. **Iris forceps** (Fig. 3.10). These are used to catch the iris for the purpose of iridectomy during operations for cataract, glaucoma, optical iridectomy and excision for iris prolapse.

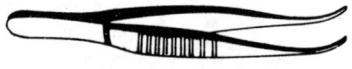

Fig. 3.10.

6. **Arruga's intracapsular (capsule holding) forceps** (Fig. 3.11). It is used to hold the lens capsule during capsule forceps method of lens delivery in intracapsular cataract extraction.

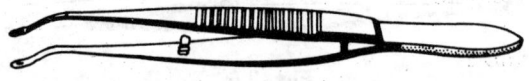

Fig. 3.11.

7. **Epilation forceps** (Fig. 3.12). These are used to epilate the cilia in trichiasis.

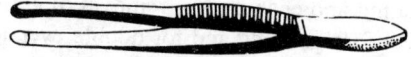

Fig. 3.12.

8. **Artery (haemostatic) forceps** (Fig. 3.13). *Uses* : (i) To catch the bleeding vessels during operations of the lids and lacrimal sac. (ii) To hold the skin and muscle stay sutures. (iii) To hold small 'pea-nut' gauze pellets for blunt dissection in lacrimal sac surgery and other extraocular surgery.

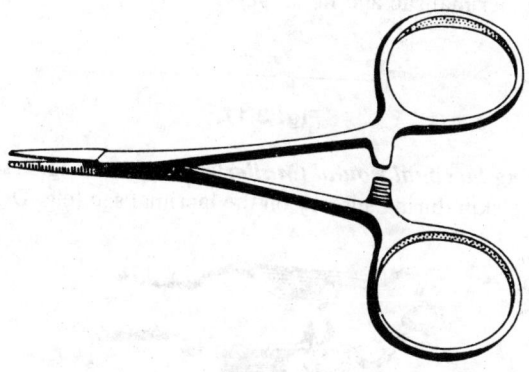

Fig. 3.13.

III. Hooks and retractors

1. **Lens expressor (hook)** (Fig. 3.14). *Uses* : (i) It is event to apply pressure on the limbus at the 6 O'clock position during the delivery of lens in intracapsular cataract extraction with Smith's (tumbling) and capsule forceps techniques and (ii) to express the nucleus in extracapsular cataract extraction.

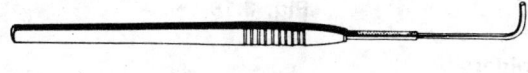

Fig. 3.14.

2. **Muscle (strabismus) hook** (Fig. 3.15). It is used to engage the extraocular muscles during surgery for squint, enucleation, and retinal detachment.

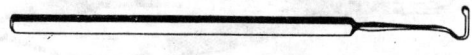

Fig. 3.15.

3. *Desmarre's retractor* (Fig. 3.16). It is used to retract the lids during examination of the eyeball in cases of blepharospasm in children, in cases with marked swelling and ecchymosis, removal of corneoscleral sutures, removal of corneal foreign body and for double eversion of upper lid to examine the superior fornix.

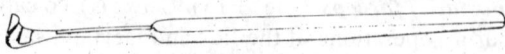

Fig. 3.16.

4. *Cat's paw lacrimal wound retractor* (Fig. 3.17). It is used to retract the skin during lacrimal sac and lid surgery.

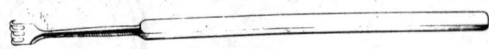

Fig. 3.17.

5. *Self-retaining lacrimal wound (Muller's) retractor* (Fig. 3.18). It is used to retract the skin during surgery on the lacrimal sac (e.g. DCT or DCR).

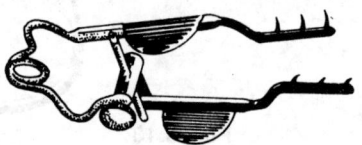

Fig. 3.18.

6. *Iris retractor* (Fig. 3.19). It is used to retract the upper edge of pupil in cryoextraction technique of ICCE.

Fig. 3.19.

IV. Needle holders

1. *Spring action (Barraquer's type) needle holder* (Fig. 3.20). It is used for passing sutures in the conjunctiva, cornea, sclera and extraocular muscles.

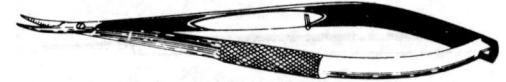

Fig. 3.20.

2. *Stevens needle holder* (Fig. 3.21) *and Arruga's needle holder.* These are very commonly used in lid surgery and for passing superior rectus suture.

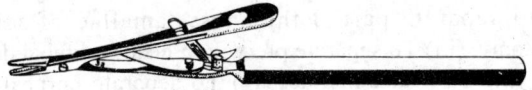

Fig. 3.21.

V. Callipers and rules

1. *Castroviejo calliper* (Fig. 3.22). It is used to take measurements during; squint, ptosis, retinal detachment and pars plana vitrectomy surgery.

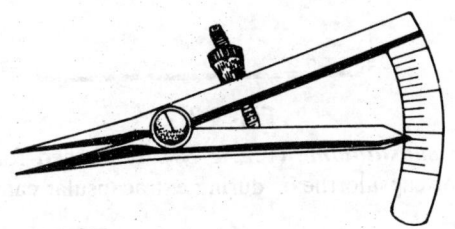

Fig. 3.22.

2. *Metallic rule:* It is used as a scale for the Castroviejo calliper for exact measurements and to measure the palpebral aperture width.

VI. Knives and knife-needles

1. *Von Graefe's knife* (Fig. 3.23). It is used for making an abinterno corneoscleral incision during cataract surgery and for iridectomy operation.

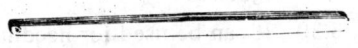

Fig. 3.23.

2. *Keratome* (Fig. 3.24). Recently keratomes are used for making self-sealing incisions for phacoemulsification.

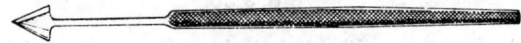

Fig. 3.24.

3. *Paracentesis needle* (Fig. 3.25). It is used for paracentesis and to make very small corneoscleral incisions.

Fig. 3.25.

4. **Tooke's knife** (Fig. 3.26). *Uses:* (i) It can be used to separate the conjunctiva and sub-conjunctival tissue from the sclera and limbus when limbal based flap is made for cataract or trabeculectomy surgery. (ii) It can also be used to separate partial thickness lamellae of sclera during trabeculectomy. (iii) To separate pterygium head or limbal dermoid from the underlying corneal lamellae. (iv) To separate corneal lamellae in lamellar keratoplasty.

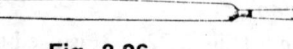

Fig. 3.26.

5. **Zeigler's knife** (Fig. 3.27). It is used for discission of after-cataract in the pupillary area.

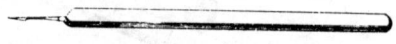

Fig. 3.27.

6. **Cystitome or capsulotome** (Fig. 3.28). It is used for doing anterior capsulotomy or capsulorrhexis during extracapsular cataract extraction.

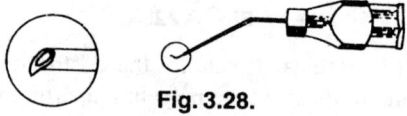

Fig. 3.28.

7. **Foreign body spud** (Fig. 3.29). It is used to remove corneal foreign body.

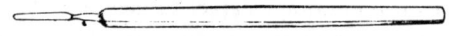

Fig. 3.29.

8. **Bowman's needle** (Fig. 3.30). It can be used for needling operation (an obsolete procedure) for congenital and traumatic cataracts in children and for after-cataract.

Fig. 3.30.

9. **Razor blade fragment with blade holder.** (Fig. 3.31) It is the most commonly used cutting device for making incisions in cataract, glaucoma, keratoplasty, sclerotomy, pterygium and many other operations.

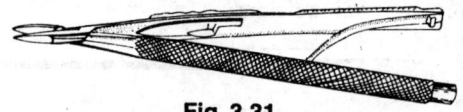

Fig. 3.31.

VII. Scissors

1. **Plain straight scissors (ringed)** (Fig. 3.32): It is used to cut conjunctiva and sutures.

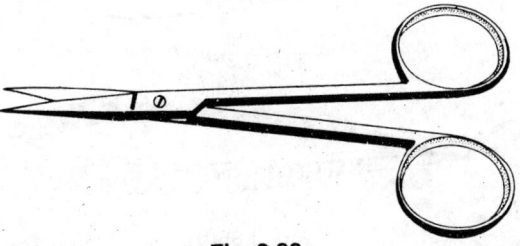

Fig. 3.32.

2. **Plain curved scissors (ringed)** (Fig. 3.33). It is used to cut and undermine conjunctiva in various operations and to undermine skin during operations on lids and lacrimal sac.

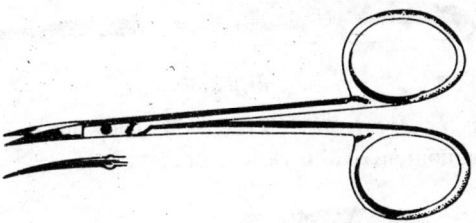

Fig. 3.33.

3. **Tenotomy scissors or strabismus scissors** (Fig. 3.34). *Uses:* (i) To cut the extraocular muscles during squint surgery and enucleation operation. (ii) To separate the delicate tissues without damaging the surrounding area in oculoplastic operations and squint surgery.

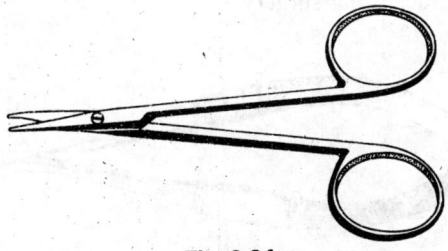

Fig. 3.34.

4. **Corneal scissors or section enlarging scissors** (Fig. 3.35). These are used to enlarge corneal or corneoscleral incision for cataract surgery and keratoplasty operation.

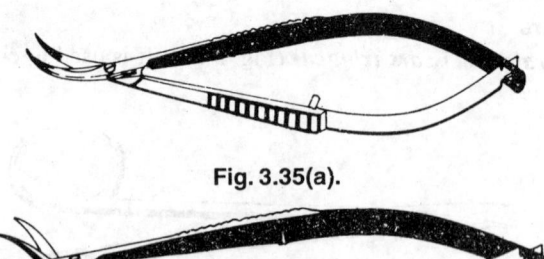

Fig. 3.35(a).

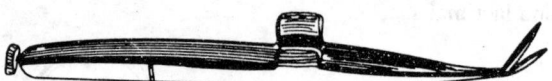

Fig. 3.35(b).

5. *de Wecker's scissors* (Fig. 3.36). It is used to perform ι idectomy, iridotomy and to cut the prolapsed formed vitreous and pupillary membrane.

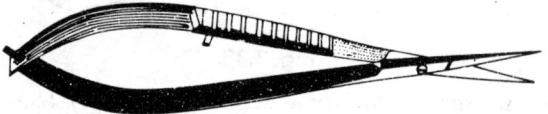

Fig. 3.36.

6. *Spring scissors (Westcott's)* (Fig. 3.37). They are used for cutting and undermining conjunctiva in various operations.

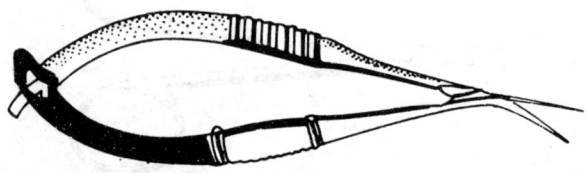

Fig. 3.37.

7. *Vannas scissors* (Fig. 3.38). These are used for cutting anterior capsule of the lens in extracapsular surgery.

Fig. 3.38.

8. *Enucleation scissors* (Fig. 3.39). They are used to cut the optic nerve during enucleation operation.

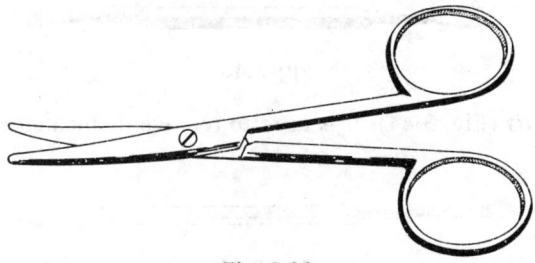

Fig. 3.39.

VIII. Clamps

1. *Lid clamp or entropion clamp* (Fig. 3.40). It is used in lid surgery e.g. entropion, and ectropion corrections. It protects the eyeball, supports the lid tissue and provides haemostasis during surgery.

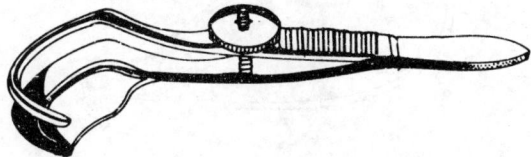

Fig. 3.40.

2. *Chalazion clamp* (Fig. 3.41). To fix the chalazion and achieve haemostasis during incision and curettage.

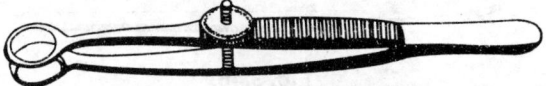

Fig. 3.41.

3. *Ptosis clamp* (Fig. 3.42). It is used to hold levator palpebrae superioris muscle during ptosis surgery.

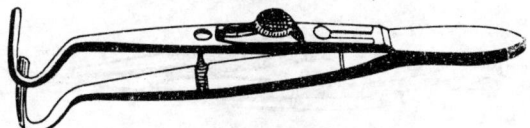

Fig. 3.42.

IX. Additional instruments for cataract surgery

1. *Lens spatula* (Fig. 3.43). It is used to apply counter-pressure at 12 O'clock position during extraction of lens in Smith's technique and expression of nucleus in extracapsular cataract extraction.

Fig. 3.43.

2. *Wire vectis* (Fig. 3.44). It is used to remove dislocated or subluxated lens.

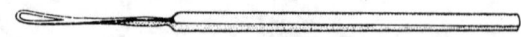

Fig. 3.44.

3. *Two-way irrigation and aspiration cannula* (Fig. 3.45). For irrigation and suction of the lens matter in extracapsular cataract extraction.

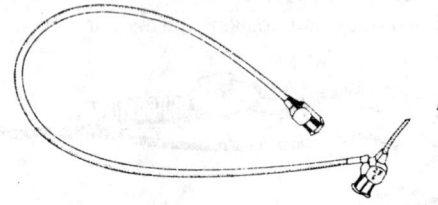

Fig. 3.45.

4. *Iris repositor* (Fig. 3.46). It is used to reposit the iris in the anterior chamber in any intraocular surgery.

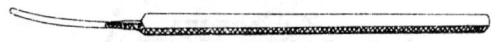

Fig. 3.46.

X. Additional instruments for intraocular lens implantation

1. *IOL holding forceps* (Fig. 3.47). It is used to hold IOL during implantation.

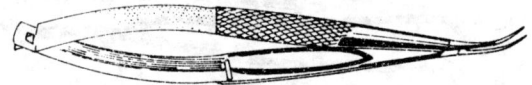

Fig. 3.47.

2. *Kelman-McPherson forceps* (Fig. 3.48) . To hold the superior haptic of IOL during placement. (ii) To tear off the anterior capsular flap in ECCE. (iii) Can be used for suture tying.

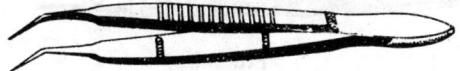

Fig. 3.48. ·

3. *IOL dialer* (Fig. 3.49). It is used to dial the IOL for proper positioning.

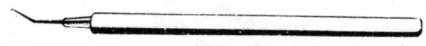

Fig. 3.49.

XI. Additional instruments for glaucoma surgery

1. *Scleral punch* (Fig. 3.50). It is used to perform punch sclerectomy during glaucoma surgery.

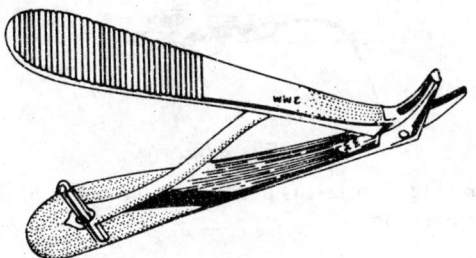

Fig. 3.50

XII. Additional instruments for lid surgery

1. *Chalazion scoop* (Fig.3.51). It is used to scoop out contents of the chalazion during incision and curettage.

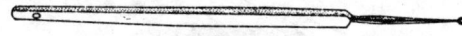

Fig. 3.51.

2. *Lid spatula* (Fig. 3.52). It is used to protect the globe and support the lid during entropion, ectropion, ptosis and other lid surgeries.

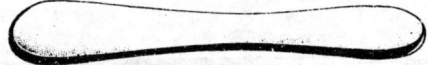

Fig. 3.52.

XIII. Additional instruments for lacrimal sac surgery (DCT and DCR)

1. *Punctum dilator (Nettleship's)* (Fig. 3.53). It is used to dilate the punctum and canaliculus during syringing, probing, dacryocystography, DCT and DCR procedures.

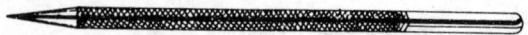

Fig. 3.53.

2. *Lacrimal probes (Bowman's)* (Fig.3.54). It is used to probe nasolacrimal duct in congenital blockage.

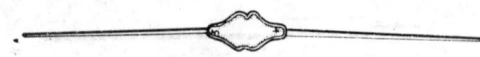

Fig. 3.54.

3. *Lacrimal cannula* (Fig. 3.55). *Uses:* (i).For syringing the lacrimal passages. (ii) As AC cannula for putting air or balanced salt solution in the anterior chamber during intraocular surgery.

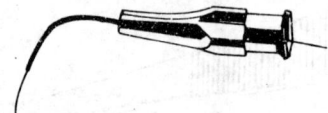

Fig. 3.55.

4. *Bone punch* (Fig. 3.56). It is used to cut the bones of the lacrimal fossa during DCR operation.

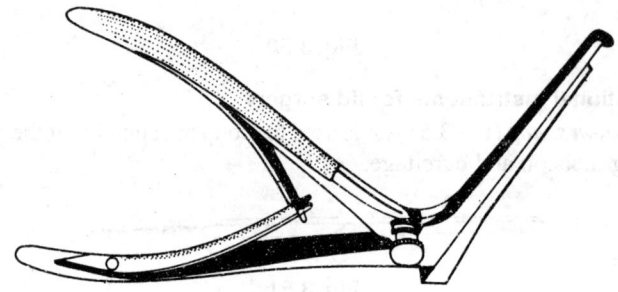

Fig. 3.56.

5. *Chisel* (Fig. 3.57). It is used to cut the bone during DCR and orbitotomy operations.

Fig. 3.57.

6. *Hammer* (Fig. 3.58). It is used to hammer the chisel during DCR and orbitotomy operations.

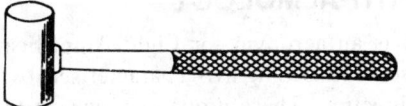

Fig. 3.58.

7. *Lacrimal sac dissector and curette* (Fig. 3.59). It is used in lacrimal sac surgery.

Fig. 3.59.

8. *Bone gouge* (Fig. 3.60). It is used to smoothen the irregularly cut margins of the bone in DCR operation.

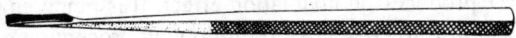

Fig. 3.60.

XIV. Additional instruments for enucleation and evisceration

1. *Optic nerve guide (enucleation spoon)* (Fig. 3.61). It is used to engage the optic nerve during enucleation.

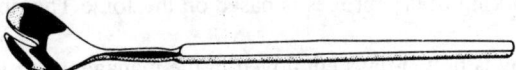

Fig. 3.61.

2. *Evisceration spatula* (Fig. 3.62). It is used to separate out the uveal tissue from the sclera during evisceration operation.

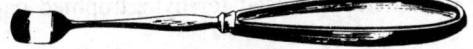

Fig. 3.62.

3. *Evisceration curette* (Fig. 3.63). It is used to curette out the intraocular contents during evisceration operation.

Fig. 3.63.

LASERS IN OPHTHALMOLOGY

The word LASER is an acronym for Light Amplification by Stimulated Emission of Radiation. Laser light is characterised by monochromaticity, coherence and collimation. These properties make it the brightest existing light.

Laser is presently used in the management of various ocular disorders. A nurse need to be familiar with laser treatment modality. A few important type of lasers and their ophthalmic uses are as below:

- *Argon laser, diode laser and* diode pumped frequency doubled YAG laser produce photocoagulation. These are used in the management of:
  - Diabetic retinopathy
  - Eales' disease
  - Small intraocular tumours etc.
- *Nd -YAG laser* produces cutting effect by photodisruption and is used for *posterior capsulotomy* in patient with thin membranous after-cataract.
- *Excimer laser* produces photoablation effect. It is being employed in the laser treatment of refractive error by following procedures :
  - Photorefractive keratectomy (PRK)
  - Laser assisted in-situ keratomileusis (LASIK).

CRYOTHERAPY IN OPHTHALMOLOGY

Cryopexy means to produce tissue injury by application of intense cold (−40°C to −100°C). This is achieved with the help of cryoprobe from a cryounit (Fig. 3.2). Working of cryoprobes is based on the Joule Thompson principle of cooling.

Cryotherapy is now-a-days employed in the management of various ocular disorders. A nurse needs to be familiar with this modality of therapy.

Uses

1. *Lids.* Cryosurgery may be used for following lesions: (i) Cryolysis for trichiasis, (ii) Cryotherapy for warts and molluscum contagiosum, (iii) Cryotherapy for basal cell carcinoma and hemangioma.
2. *Conjunctiva.* Cryotherapy is used for hypertrophied papillae of vernal catarrh.
3. *Cornea.* Herpes simplex keratitis may be treated by cryotherapy.
4. *Lens.* Cryoextraction of the lens is the best intracapsular technique. It is the most common use of cryo in developing countries.
5. *Cliary body.* Cyclocryopexy for absolute glaucoma and neovascular glaucoma.
6. *Retina.* (i) Cryopexy is widely used for sealing retinal holes in retinal detachment. (ii) Prophylactic cryopexy to prevent retinal detachment in certain prone cases. (iii) Retinal cryopexy for neovascularization. (iv) Cryotreatment of retinoblastoma and angioma.

4

Optics and
Errors of Refraction

LIGHT

Light is the visible portion of the electromagnetic radiation spectrum. It lies between ultraviolet and infrared portions, from 400 nm at the violet end of the spectrum to 700 nm at the red end. The white light consists of seven colours denoted by VIBGYOR (violet, indigo, blue, green, yellow, orange and red).

Light ray is the term used to describe the radius of the concentric wave forms. A group of parallel rays of light is called a *beam of light*.

Some important points to remember about light rays are as follows :

- The media of the eye are uniformally permeable to the visible rays between 600 nm and 390 nm.
- Cornea absorbs rays shorter than 295 nm. Therefore, rays between 600 nm and 295 nm only can reach the lens.
- Lens absorbs rays shorter than 350 nm. Therefore, rays between 600 and 350 nm can reach the retina in phakic eye; and those between 600 nm and 295 nm in aphakic eyes.

GEOMETRICAL OPTICS

The behaviour of light rays is determined by ray-optics. A ray of light is the straight line path followed by light in-going from one point to another. The ray-optics, therefore, uses the geometry of straight lines to account for the macroscopic phenomena like rectilinear propagation, reflection and refraction. That is why the ray-optics is also called geometrical optics.

The knowledge of geometrical optics is essential to understand the optics of eye, errors of refraction and their correction. Therefore, some of its important aspects are described in the following text.

Reflection of light

Reflection of light is a phenomenon of change in the path of light rays without any change in the medium (Fig. 4.1). The light rays falling on a

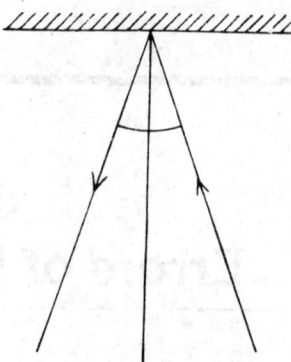

Fig. 4.1. Laws of reflection.

reflecting surface are called *incident rays* and those reflected by it are *reflected rays*. A line drawn at right angle to the surface is called the normal. The *laws of reflection* are :

1. The incident ray, the reflected ray and the normal at the point of incident, all lie in the same plane.
2. The angle of incidence is equal to the angle of reflection.

Refraction of light

Refraction of light is the phenomenon of change in the path of light, when it goes from one medium to another. The basic cause of refraction is change in the velocity of light in going from one medium to the other. The *laws of refraction* are (Fig. 4.2):

1. The incident and refracted rays are on opposite sides of the normal and all the three are in the same plane.

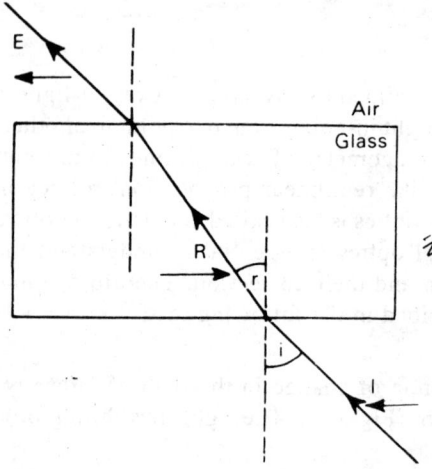

Fig. 4.2. Laws of refraction. N1 and N2 (normals); I (incident ray); i (angle of incidence); R (refracted ray, bent towards normal); r (angle of refraction); E (emergent ray, bent away from the normal).

2. The ratio of sine of angle of incidence to the sine of angle of refraction is constant for the part of media in contact. This constant is denoted by the letter n and is called *'refractive index'* of the medium 2 in which the refracted ray lies with respect to medium 1 (in which the incident ray lies), i.e. $\frac{\sin i}{\sin r} = {}^{1}n_{2}$. When the medium 1 is air (or vacuum), then n is called the refractive index of the medium 2. This law is also called *Snell's law of refraction.*

Total internal reflection

When a ray of light travelling from an optically denser medium to an optically rarer medium is incident at an angle greater than the critical angle of the pair of media in contact, the ray is totally reflected back into the denser medium (Fig. 4.3). This phenomenon is called total *internal reflection.*

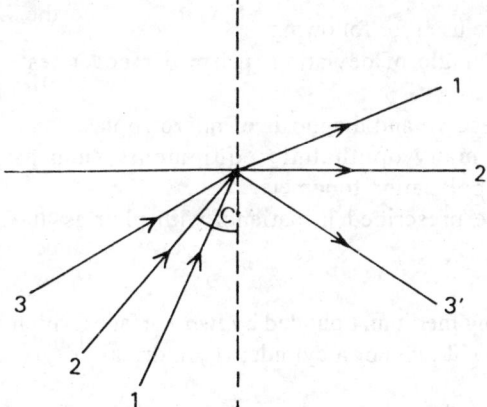

Fig. 4.3. Showing (1-1) refraction of light; (2-2) path of refracted ray at critical angle, c; (3-3) total internal reflection.

The *critical angle* refers to the angle of incidence in the denser medium, corresponding to which angle of refraction in the rare medium is 90°. It is represented by C and its value depends on the nature of media in contact.

The principle of total internal reflection is utilized in many optical equipments; such as fibroptic lights, applanation tonometer, and gonioscope.

Prism

A prism is a refracting medium, having two plane surfaces, inclined at an angle. The greater the angle formed by two surfaces at the apex, the stronger the prismatic effect. The prism produces displacement of the objects seen through it towards apex (away from the base) (Fig. 4.4). The power of a prism is measured in prism dioptres. One prism dioptre (Δ)

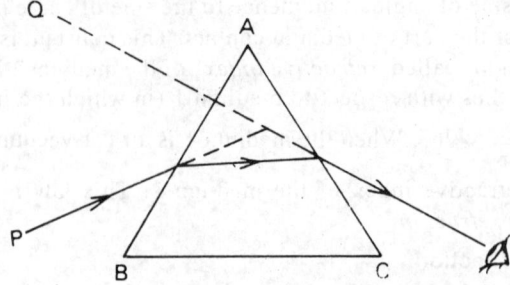

Fig. 4.4. Refraction by a prism.

produces displacement of an object by one cm when kept at a distance of one metre. Two prism dioptres of displacement is approximately equal to one degree of arc.

Uses

In ophthalmology, prisms are used for following:

1. Objective measurement of angle of deviation (prism bar cover test, Krimsky test).
2. Measurement of fusional reserve and diagnosis of microtropia.
3. Prisms are also used in many ophthalmic equipments such as gonioscope, keratometer, applanation tonometer.
4. Therapeutically, prisms are prescribed in patients with phorias and diplopia.

Lenses

A lens is a transparent refracting medium, bounded by *two* surfaces which form a part of a sphere (spherical lens) or a cylinder (cylindrical or toric lens).

Cardinal data of a lens (Fig. 4.5):

1. *Centre of curvature* (C) of the spherical lens is the centre of the sphere of which the refracting lens surface is a part.

2. *Radius of curvature* of the spherical lens is the radius of the sphere of which the refracting surface is a part.

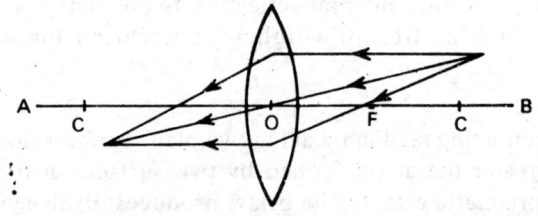

Fig. 4.5. Cardinal points of a convex lens, optical centre (O); principal focus (F); centre of curvature (C) and principal axis (AB).

3. *The principal axis* (AB) of the lens is the line joining the centres of curvatures of its surfaces.

4. *Optical centre* (O) of the lens corresponds to the nodal point of a thick lens. It is a point on the principal axis in the lens, the rays passing from where do not undergo deviation. In meniscus lenses the optical centre lies outside the lens.

5. *The principal focus* (F) of a lens is that point on the principal axis where parallel rays of light, after passing through the lens, converge (in convex lens) or appear to diverge (in concave lens).

6. *The focal length* (*f*) of a lens is the distance between the optical centre and the principal focus.

7. *Power of a lens* (P) is defined as the ability of the lens to converge a beam of light falling on the lens. For a converging (convex) lens the power is taken as positive and for a diverging (concave) lens power is taken as negative. It is measured as reciprocal of the focal length in metres i.e. $P = \dfrac{1}{f}$ The unit of power is dioptre (D). One dioptre is the power of a lens of focal length one metre.

Types of lenses

Lenses are of two types: the spherical and cylindrical (or toric or astigmatic).

1. Spherical lenses. Spherical lenses are bounded by two spherical surfaces and are mainly of two types convex and concave.

(i) **Convex lens** or plus lens is a converging lens. It may be of biconvex, plano-convex or concavo-convex (meniscus) type (Fig. 4.6).

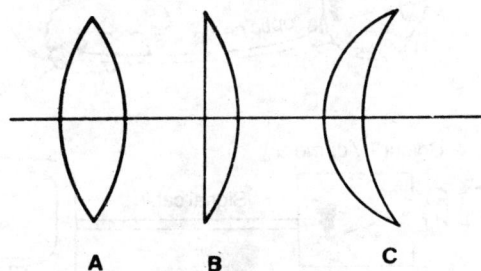

Fig. 4.6. Basic forms of a convex lens: (A) biconvex; (B) plano-convex; (C) concavo-convex.

(ii) **Concave lens** or minus lens is a diverging lens. It is of three types: biconcave, plano-concave and convexo-concave (meniscus) (Fig. 4.7).

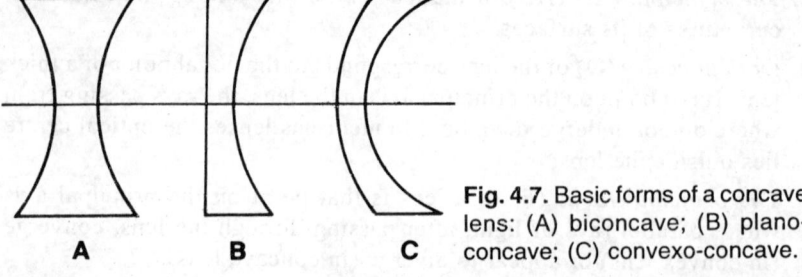

Fig. 4.7. Basic forms of a concave lens: (A) biconcave; (B) plano-concave; (C) convexo-concave.

2. Cylindrical lens. A cylindrical lens acts only in one axis i.e. power is incorporated in one axis, the other axis having zero power. A cylindrical lens may be convex (plus) or concave (minus).

OPTICS OF THE EYE

As an optical instrument the eye is well compared to a camera with retina acting as a unique kind of film. The focussing system of the eye is composed of several refracting structures which include cornea, aqueous humour, crystalline lens and the vitreous humour. The total diopteric power of the eye is about +60 D; out of which about +44 D is contributed by cornea and +16 D by the crystalline lens.

The functioning of the eye as an optical instrument can be considered to be analogous to a closed circuit colour TV system (Fig. 4.8)

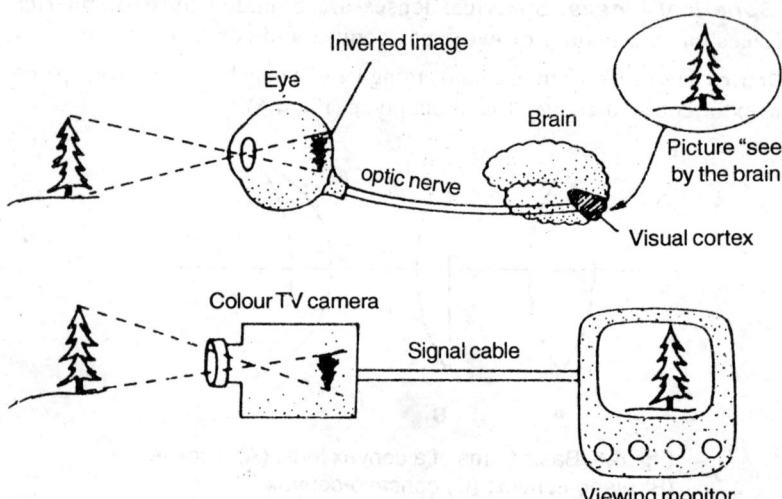

Fig. 4.8. The sense of sight is in many ways similar to a closed circuit colour TV system. It is superior in all respects except ease of replacement.

Reduced Eye. *The optics of eye otherwise is very complex. However, for understanding, Listing has simplified the data by choosing single principal and nodal point. This is called Listing's reduced eye. The simplified data of this eye (Fig. 4.9) are as follows :*

- The principal point (P) lies 1.5 mm behind the anterior surface of cornea.
- The nodal point (N) is situated 7.2 mm behind the anterior surface of cornea.
- The anterior focal point is 15.7 mm in front of the anterior surface of cornea.
- The posterior focal point (on the retina) is 24.4 mm behind the anterior surface of cornea.
- The anterior focal length is 17.2 mm (15.7 + 1.5) and posterior focal length is 22.9 mm (24.4 – 1.5).

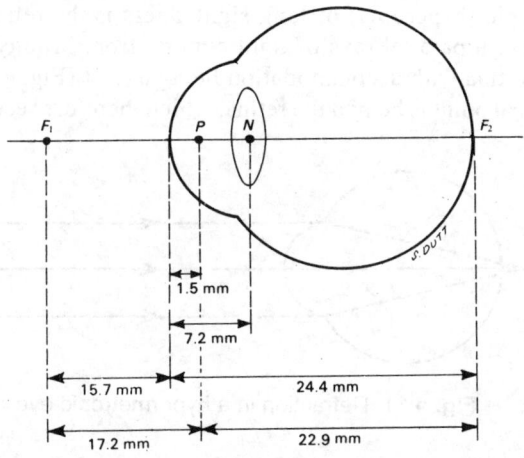

Fig. 4.9. Cardinal points of (a) normal eye; (b) reduced eye.

ERRORS OF REFRACTION

EMMETROPIA

Emmetropia (optically normal eye) can be defined as a state of refraction, when the parallel rays of light coming from infinity are focussed at the sensitive layer of retina with the accommodation being at rest (Fig. 4.10).

AMETROPIA

Ametropia (a condition of refractive error), is defined as a state of refraction, when the parallel rays of light coming from infinity, (with

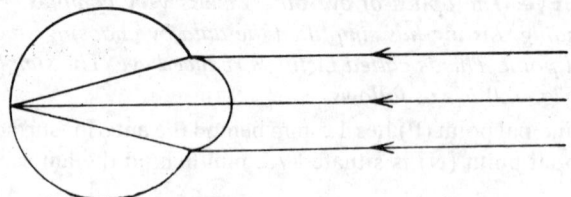

Fig. 4.10. Refraction in an emmetropic eye.

accommodation at rest), are focussed either in front or behind the sensitive layer of retina, in one or both the meridians. The ametropia includes myopia, hypermetropia and astigmatism.

HYPERMETROPIA

Hypermetropia (hyperopia) or long sightedness is the refractive state of the eye wherein parallel rays of light coming from infinity are focussed behind the retina with accommodation being at rest (Fig. 4.11). Thus the posterior focal point is behind the retina, which therefore receives a blurred image.

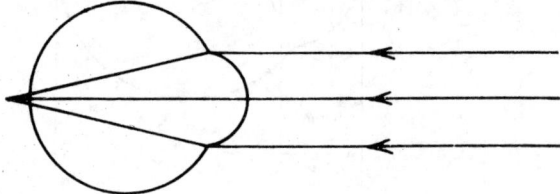

Fig. 4.11. Refraction in a hypermetropic eye.

Etiology

1. *Axial hypermetropia* is by far the commonest form. It occurs due to short axial length of the eyeball.
2. *Curvatural hypermetropia* occurs due to comparatively flatter curvature of the cornea or lens or both.
3. *Index hypermetropia* results due to change in the refractive index of the lens.
4. *Absence of the lens* (aphakia) either congenital or acquired (following surgical removal of the lens) leads to high hypermetropia.

Clinical features

Hypermetropia patients, depending upon the degree of hypermetropia and age of the patient may suffer from following symptoms :

1. *Asthenopic symptoms* occur due to constant use of accommodation. These include tiredness of eyes, frontal or frontotemporal headache,

watering and mild photophobia. These asthenopic symptoms are especially associated with near work and increase towards evening.

2. *Defective vision.* When the degree of hypermetropia is more (which cannot be fully corrected by accommodation) patient may have difficulty in near vision or both near and far vision.

Treatment

1. *Glasses and contact lenses.* Hypermetropia can be corrected by appropriate convex lenses in the form of spectacles or contact lenses after meticulous refraction.

2. *Refractive corneal surgery.* Hypermetropia can also be treated by changing the corneal curvature with excimer laser.

MYOPIA

Myopia or short-sightedness is a type of refractive error in which parallel rays of light coming from infinity are focussed in front of the retina when accommodation is at rest (Fig. 4.12). Defective vision for distance (short sightedness) is the main symptom of myopia. In myopic patients eyes are usually prominent with large pupils and deep anterior chamber.

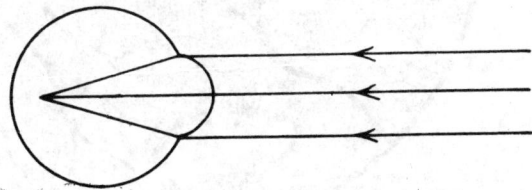

Fig. 4.12. Refraction in a myopic eye.

Etiology

1. *Axial myopia* results from increase in the antero-posterior length of the eyeball.

2. *Curvatural myopia* occurs due to increased curvature of the cornea, lens or both.

3. *Index myopia* results from increase in the refractive index of the crystalline lens associated with nuclear sclerosis.

Clinical types

1. *Congenital myopia* is present since birth. Usually the error is of about −8 to − 10 diopters, which mostly remains constant. It may be associated with other ocular congenital anomalies.

2. *Simple myopia.* It is the commonest variety, which results from normal biological variation in the development of eye. Simple myopia starts

at school age and very slowly progresses till adult age. Usually the error does not exceed −6 to −8 diopters.

3. **Pathological myopia or degenerative myopia** is a rapidly progressive error resulting in high myopia (more than −8 D) during early adult life, which is usually associated with degenerative changes in the retina (Fig. 4.13, PL.I.1). Genetic factors play major role in the etiology of pathological myopia.

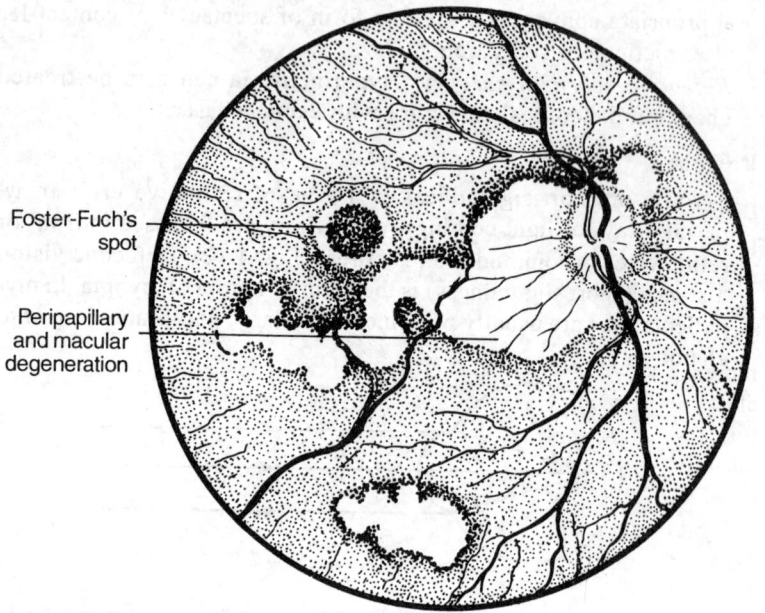

Foster-Fuch's spot

Peripapillary and macular degeneration

Fig. 4.13. Fundus changes in pathological myopia.

Treatment

1. **Optical treatment** consists of prescribing appropriate concave lenses in the form of glasses or contact lenses.

2. **Refractive corneal surgery** for myopia is very effective and includes the following :

   i. *Radial keratotomy.* Its basic principal is to decrease the curvature of cornea by performing radial incisions.

   ii. *Photo-refractive keratectomy (PRK).* It is performed with excimer laser. It is more safe than radial keratotomy.

   iii. *Laser assisted in situ keratomileusis (LASIK).* It is best available refractive corneal surgery .

ASTIGMATISM

Astigmatism is a type of refractive error wherein the refraction varies in the different meridia of the eye. Consequently, the ray of light entering in the eye cannot converge to a point focus but form focal lines.

Etiology. Astigmatism, usually occurs due to unequal curvature of cornea. Rarely it may occur due to subluxation abnormalities of the curvature of the lens.

Types : Astigmatism is of following types :

1. *Regular astigmatism* is present when the two principal meridians are at right angles. It can be simple, compound or mixed.
2. *Irregular astigmatism* occurs when the corneal surface is irregular.

Treatment. Regular astigmatism can be treated by cylindrical lenses in the form of spectacles or contact lenses. Irregular astigmatism cannot be treated by spectacles. Contact lenses or keratoplasty may be needed for irregular astigmatism.

PRESBYOPIA

Presbyopia (eyesight of old age) is not an error of refraction, but a condition of physiological insufficiency of accommodation, leading to failing vision for near. It usually occurs after 40 years of age.

Etiology. Decrease in the accommodative power of crystalline lens with increasing age, leading to presbyopia occur due to : (i) decrease in the elasticity and plasticity of the crystalline lens (which results from age related sclerosis), and (2) age related decrease in the power of ciliary muscle.

Clinical features. Typically patient complains of slowly progressive difficulty in focussing the near objects, whilst distant vision is not affected.

Treatment. Convex glasses of an appropriate power depending upon the age of the patient are required for near work.

DETERMINATION OF REFRACTIVE ERRORS

The procedure of determining and correcting refractive error is termed as *refraction.* It is an art that can only be mastered by practice. The refraction comprises two complementary methods, the objective and subjective.

Objective methods include retinoscopy. auto-refractometry and kerotometry. Subjective refraction is the technique of finding out acceptance of glasses by the patient.

RETINOSCOPY

Retinoscopy also termed as *skiascopy* or *shadow test* is an objective method of finding out the error of refraction by the technique of neutralization.

Principle. It is based on the fact that when light is reflected from a mirror into the eye, the direction in which the light travels across the pupil will depend upon the refractive state of the eye.

Cycloplegia in retinoscopy are used in children and young hypermetropia where accommodation is likely to hinder the exact retinoscopy. *Atropine* (1% ointment 3 times a day for 3 days) is preferred in children below 8 years of age. *Homatropine* (2%) and *cycloplentolate* (1%) are sufficient in older children and young adults.

Prerequisites for retinoscopy

1. *A dark room,* preferably 6 metre long, or which can be converted into 6 metres by use of a plane mirror.
2. *A trial box* containing spherical and cylindrical lenses of variable plus and minus powers, a pinhole, an occluder and prisms.
3. *A trial frame* (Fig. 4.14) preferably of adjustable type which can be used in children as well as adults.

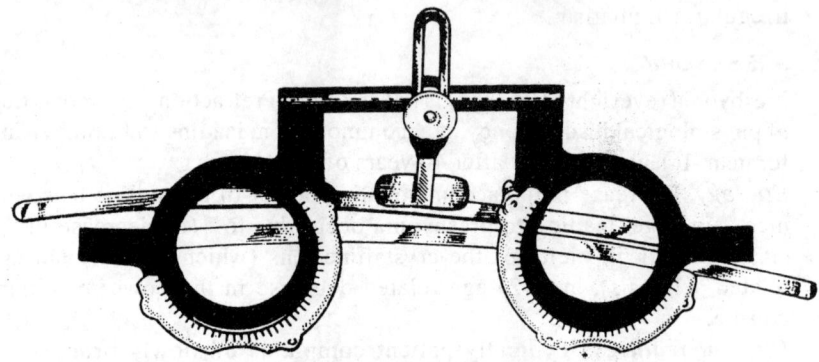

Fig. 4.14. Trial frame.

4. *Vision box.* A Snellen's self-illuminated vision box (Fig. 4.15).

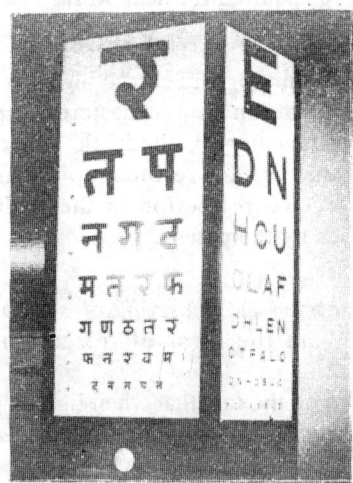

Fig. 4.15. Snellen's vision box.

5. *Retinoscope* is a simple device to perform the retinoscopy. Broadly, retinoscopes available are of two types:

(a) *Mirror retinoscopes* are cheap and the most commonly employed. A source of light is required when using mirror retinoscope, which is kept above and behind the head of the patient. A mirror retinoscope may consist of a single plane mirror (Fig. 4.16a) or a combination of plane and concave mirrors (*Pristley-Smith mirror*– Fig. 4.16b).

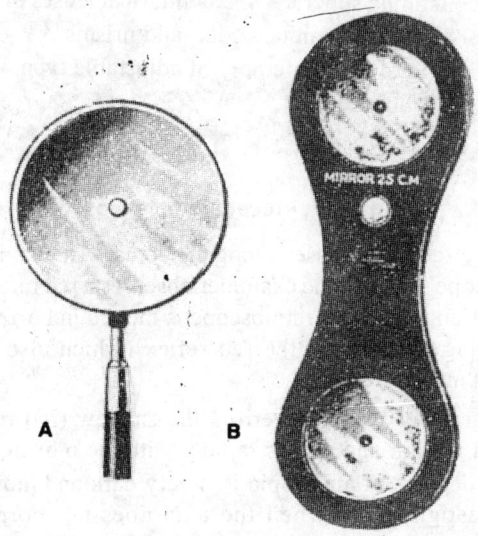

Fig. 4.16. Mirror retinoscopes: (A) plane mirror;
(B) Pristley's Smith mirror.

(b) *Self-illuminated retinoscopes* are costly but handy. Two types of self-illuminated retinoscopes available are: a spot retinoscope and a streak retinoscope. The streak retinoscope is more popular. In it the usual circular beam of light is modified to produce a linear streak of light by using a plano-cylindrical retinoscopy mirror. The steak retinoscopy is more sensitive than spot retinoscopy in detecting astigmatism.

In practice, plane mirror is used for retinoscopy. In patients with hazy media and high degree of ametropia concave mirror is more useful.

Procedure
The patient is made to sit at a distance of 1 metre from the examiner (Fig. 4.17). With the help of a retinoscope, light is thrown onto the patient's eye, who is instructed to look at a far point (to relax the accommodation). However, when a cycloplegic has been used, the patient can look directly into the light

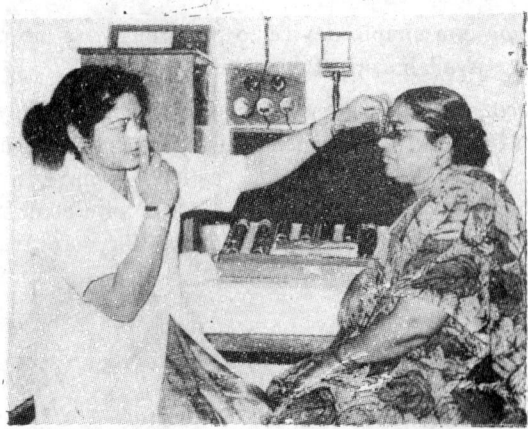

Fig. 4.17. Procedure of retinoscopy.

and have the refraction assessed along the actual visual axis. Through a hole in the retinoscope's mirror, the examiner observes a red reflex in the pupillary area of the patient. Then the retinoscope is moved in horizontal and vertical meridia keeping a watch on the red reflex (which also moves when the retinoscope is moved).

In low degrees of refractive errors the shadow (red reflex) seen in the pupillary area is faint and moves rapidly with the movement of the mirror; while in high degrees of ametropia it is very dark and moves slowly. In the presence of astigmatism, when the axis does not correspond with the movement of the mirror, the shadow appears to swirl round.

Observations and inferences. Depending upon the movement of the red reflex when a plane mirror retinoscope is used at a distance of 1 metre) the results are interpreted as below:

1. No movement of red reflex indicates myopia of 1 D.
2. When red reflex moves along with the movement of the retinoscope, it indicates either emmetropia or hypermetropia or myopia of less than 1 dioptre.
3. A movement of red reflex against the movement of the retinoscope implies myopia of more than 1 dioptre.

Autorefractometry

Autorefractometry is an objective method of finding error of refraction using a computerized autorefractometer. This technique quickly gives information about the refractive error of the patient in terms of sphere, cylinder with axis and inter-pupillary distance. It is a good alternative to retinoscopy in busy practice. Subjective verification is must even after autorefractometry.

Subjective refraction

Subjective refraction is meant for finding out the most suitable lenses to be prescribed. When performed after cycloplegic retinoscopy, it is termed as post-mydriatic test (PMT). PMT should be done after 3 days when cyclopentolate or homatropine is used and after 3 weeks when atropine is used.

Subjective refraction is carried out separately for each eye. The appropriate lenses found by the retinoscopy are inserted in the trial frame and most suitable lenses are found by increasing and decreasing the power of lenses. The subjective refraction should be verified using duochrome test, astigmatic far test or Jackson's cross cylinder test.

The correction for near vision by additional convex spherical lenses is usually required in patients above 40 years of age.

CONTACT LENSES

Contact lens is a thin lens of the corneal curvature which is put on the cornea by the patient. Contact lenses are so named since they are in direct contact with the outer surface of the eye. Thus, the front surface of a contact lens replaces the anterior surface of cornea. Therefore, in addition to correction of refractive error, the irregularities of the front surface of cornea can also be corrected by the contact lens.

Parts of a contact lens are shown in Fig. 4.18

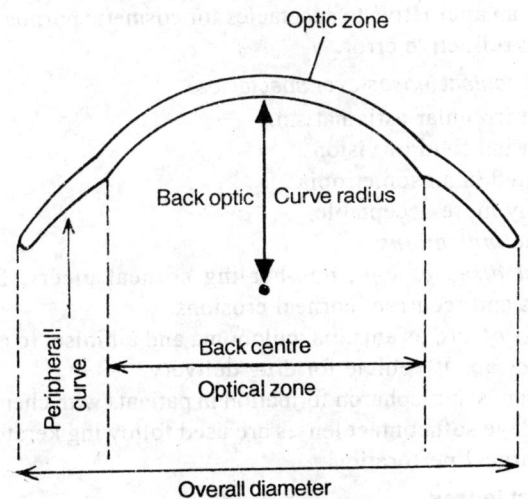

Fig. 4.18. A contact lens.

Types of contact lenses

1. *Hard Lenses.* These are made of PMMA (Polymethylmethacrylate) and are usually 8.5 to 10 mm in diameter.

Advantages. The PMMA has a high optical quality, light in weight, nontoxic, durable and cheap.

Disadvantages. PMMA is practically impermeable to O_2 so chances of corneal hypoxia and oedema are always there. Being hard, it can cause corneal abrasions.

2. *Gas permeable (GP) lenses.* These are made up of a mixture of hard and soft material (e.g. copolymes of PMMA and silicone), which is permeable to O_2. Basically these lenses are also hard, but, some how due to their O_2 permeability they have become popular by the name of *semisoft lenses.*

Advantages. Good O_2 permeability and so no corneal hypoxia.

Disadvantages. Scratch and break more easily than the PMMA lenses.

3. *Soft lenses.* These are made up of HEMA (hydroxyethyl methacrylate). These are made about 1-2 mm larger than the corneal diameter.

Advantages. Being soft and oxygen permeable, they are most comfortable and so well tolerated.

Disadvantages include problem of wettability, proteinaceous deposits,getting cracked, limited life, inferior optical quality and more chances of corneal infections.

Indications of contact lens use

1. *Optical indications* include anisometropia, unilateral aphakia, high myopia, keratoconus and irregular astigmatism. However, contact lenses can be used as an alternative to spectacles for cosmetic purposes, by every patient having refractive error.

Advantages of contact lenses over spectacles

- Can correct irregular astigmatism.
- Provide normal field of vision
- Well tolerated in anisometropia
- Cosmetically more acceptable.

2. *Therapeutic indications*

   i. *Corneal diseases* e.g., non-healing corneal ulcers, filamentary keratitis and recurrent corneal erosions.

   ii. *Diseases of iris,* as aniridia, coloboma and albinism to avoid glare.

   iii. *In glaucoma,* as vehicle for drug delivery.

   iv. To prevent symblepharon formation in patients with chemical burns.

   v. As bandage soft contact lenses are used following keratoplasty and microcorneal perforation.

Care of contact lenses

Careful and meticulous attention to contact lens hygeine is required to be paid, as the risks associated with their use are of paramount significance. An ophthalmic staff nurse should give the following instructions to contact lens users:

1. Hands should be thoroughly cleaned before handling the contact lenses.
2. On removal of contact lens, proper surface care of contact lens with a surfactant cleaner should be done. The surfactant removes deposits, debris and microbial biofilm.
3. Liberal rinsing of contact lens with preserved or non-preserved <u>sterile</u> saline.
4. Contact lens should be disinfected with appropriate system. Hard and rigid gas permeable lenses are treated with chemical disinfection only, as these cannot withstand heating. Soft contact lenses may be disinfected using either a thermal or chemical system.
5. Before insertion, the contact lenses should be rinsed again with sterile saline.
6. Enzyme cleaning should be done every week. Enzymes are specific catalysts which help to remove lens proteins. Thorough rinsing of contact lenses with sterile saline should be done after ezyme cleaning, as few enzymes like papain may be sensitizing to some individuals.
7. Multipurpose solutions are available in the market which can be used for soaking, cleaning, disinfecting and rinsing of contact lenses.
8. Patients should not sleep (except with extended wear lenses) or swim with their contact lenses on.

Insertion and removal of contact lenses

After teaching care and handling of contact lenses, a staff nerve is supposed to train the patient in insertion and removal of contact lenses.

Insertion

Technique1 (Fig. 4.19A). Place the wet lens hollow side up on the end of the middle finger of your right hand just above and toward the middle of the margin of your right lower lid. Pull your lower lid down and hold it firmly against the bone below it. Bring your left hand over your head and place the forefinger or middle finger just below and toward the middle of the margin of your right upper lid. Pull your upper lid up and hold it firmly against the bone above it. Insert the lens. To insert the lens on your left eye, your hands may be used the same way or you may alternate your hands.

Technique 2 (Fig.4.19B). Spread the forefinger and middle finger of your right hand in the form of an open pair of scissors. Hold the right lower lid down with the middle finger, and hold the right upper lid up with the forefinger. Place the wet lens with its concave or hollow side up on the forefinger of your left hand. This finger is held relatively parallel to the ground and the lens is inserted. To insert the lens on your left eye your hand may be used the same way or you may alternate your hands.

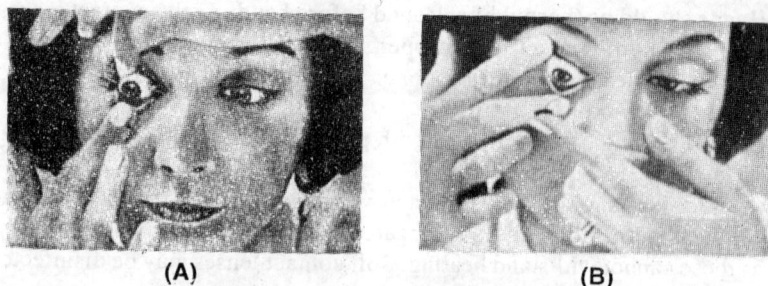

(A) (B)

Fig. 4.19. Techniques of contact lens insertion.

Removal

Technique 1 (Fig. 4.20A). Bend over so your head is relatively parallel to the floor. Cup your left hand under your right eye. Place the thumb, index or forefinger of your right hand at the outer corner of your eyelids. Look straight down and open both eyes wide. Pull the finger in an upward and outward direction. If the lens does not come out, it may be necessary to blink simultaneously while pulling. The opposite hands are used for the left eye.

Technique 2 (Fig. 4.20B). Bend over so your head is relatively parallel to the floor. Place the middle finger of your right hand along the right lower lid margin and the forefinger of your right hand along the right upper lid margin. Cup your left hand under your right eye to catch the lens. Draw your lids away from the lens, hold them tightly against the eye, and press them tightly together while looking straight ahead. An alternate method is to pull both lids to the side with the forefinger on the lower lid and the middle finger on the upper lid, or with the thumb on the lower lid and the forefinger on the upper lid. The opposite hands are used for the left eye.

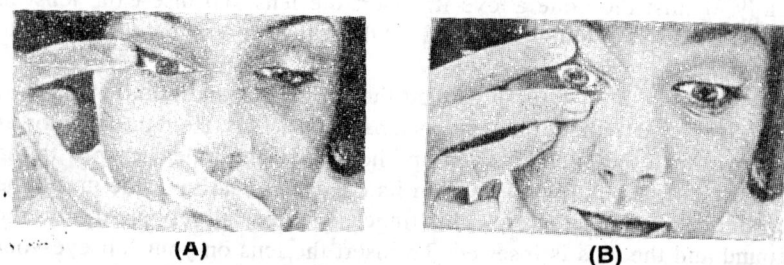

(A) (B)

Fig. 4.20. Technique of contact lens removal.

5

Diseases of Conjunctiva

CONJUNCTIVITIS

Inflammation of the conjunctiva (conjunctivitis) is classically defined as conjunctival hyperaemia associated with a discharge which may be watery, mucoid, mucopurulent or purulent.

Classification

1. *Infective conjunctivitis*

   ~ Acute
   1 Acute mucopurulent conjunctivitis
   2. Ophthalmia neonatorum
   3. Acute viral conjunctivitis
   4. Adult inclusion conjunctivitis

   Subacute or chronic
   1. Chronic simple conjunctivitis
   2. Angular conjunctivitis
   3. Trachoma

2. *Allergic conjunctivitis*
   1. Simple allergic conjunctivitis
   2. Spring catarrh
   3. Phlyctenular conjunctivitis

INFECTIVE CONJUNCTIVITIS

ACUTE MUCOPURULENT CONJUNCTIVITIS

It is the most common type of acute bacterial conjunctivitis characterized by marked conjunctival hyperaemia and mucopurulent discharge from the eye.

Etiology

Predisposing factors for bacterial conjunctivitis are poor hygiene, hot dry climate and poor sanitation. It is contagious and spreads by flies, fingers and fomites.

Common causative bacteria are *Staphylococcus aureus, Haemophilus influenzae* (Koch-Weeks bacillus), *Pneumococcus* and *Streptococcus pyogenase.*

Clinical features

Mucopurulent conjunctivitis is usually bilateral and a self-limiting disease. It is characterized by following symptoms and signs.

Symptoms

- Discomfort and grittiness in eyes
- Redness
- Mucopurulent discharge and crusting
- Sticking together of lid margins with discharge.
- Mild photophobia

Signs (Fig. 5.1 & Pl I.2)

- Conjunctival congestion, more marked in fornices is present giving the appearence of red eye.
- Chemosis i.e. swelling of the conjunctiva.
- Flakes of mucopus may be seen in the fornices, canthi and lid margins.

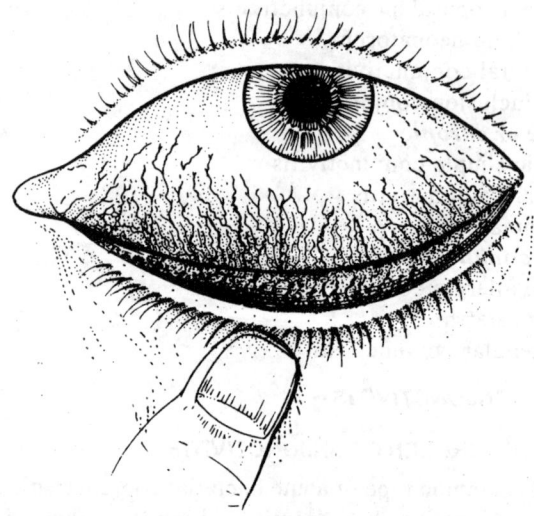

Fig. 5.1. Signs of acute mucopurulent conjunctivitis.

Complications

Occasionally the disease may be complicated by marginal corneal ulcer, superficial keratitis, blepharitis and chronic conjunctivitis.

Differential diagnosis

The three most common causes of a red eye are all seen by nurses working in the casualty department and their differential diagnosis is outlined in Table 5.1.

Table 5.1. Distinguishing features between three most common causes of red eye i.e. acute conjunctivitis, acute iridocyclitis and acute congestive glaucoma

Feature	Acute Conjunctivitis	Acute Iridocyclitis	Acute Congestive glaucoma
Pain	Grittiness	Moderate	Severe
Discharge	Mucopurulent	Watery	Watery
Vision	Good	Slightly impaired	Markedly impaired
Pupil	Normal	Constricted, may be irregular	Dilated, oral and fixed
Iris	Normal	Muddy	Oedematous
Intraocular pressure	Normal	Usually normal	Markedly raised
Constitutional symptoms	Absent	Little	Prostrations and vomiting

Treatment

1. *Topical antibiotics* to control the infection constitute the main treatment of acute mucopurulent conjunctivitis. For most effective use of antibiotics, it is desirable to obtain a conjunctival swab for culture and sensitivity testing of the infecting organism. Although routine treatment with a wide spectrum drug such as 1% choramphenicol, 0.3% gentamycin or framycetine eye drops should normally be instituted immediately. The use of antibiotic eye ointment at bed time will help to reduce the stickiness of the lids in the morning.
2. *Gentle swabbing of the lids* to remove crusts and irrigation of the conjunctival sac with saline may give same comfort.
3. *Dark goggles* reduce the photophobia.

Prophylaxis

- Avoid using the patient's towel or other fomites.
- Avoid contact with infected eye.
- Patient must keep his hands clean.

OPHTHALMIA NEONATORUM

Ophthalmia neonatorum refers to bilateral conjunctivitis occurring in an infant, less than 30 days old.

Etiology

Mode of infection. The most common mode of infection is during delivery from the infected birth canal of the mother. Infected hands of the persons handling the delivery and the soiled clothes or fingers with infected lochia are other common modes of infection.

Causative organisms are as follows :

Gonococcal infection from the mother suffering from gonorrhoea is responsible for severe form of ophthalmia neonatorum. Fortunately incidence of this blinding disease is declining due to prophylaxis and effective treatment of gonorrhoea.

Other bacterial infection responsible for ophthalmia neonatorum are staphylococcus aureus, streptococcus haemolyticus and streptococcus pneumoniae.

Neonatal inclusion conjunctivitis caused by serotypes D to K of chlamydia trachomatis is emerging as an important cause of ophthalmia neonatorum.

Herpes simplex ophthalmia neonatorum is a rare condition caused by herpes simplex-II virus.

Chemical conjunctivitis caused by silver nitrate or antibiotics used for prophylaxis is also a cause of ophthalmia neonatorum.

Clinical features

1. Neonates may be irritable or cry excessively due to pain and discomfort.
2. *Conjunctival discharge* may be mucopurulent or purulent.
3. Lids are usually swollen.
4. Conjunctiva may show hyperaemia and chemosis.

Complications

Untreated cases, especially of gonococcal ophthalmia neonatorum may develop corneal ulceration, which may perforate rapidly resulting sometimes in panophthalmitis.

Treatment

Prophylactic treatment is always better than curative treatment for ophthalmia neonatorum.

Prophylaxis

Nurses posted in maternity wards can play a major role in the antenatal, natal and postnatal care.

1. *Antenatal measures* include thorough care of mother and treatment of genital infections when suspected.
2. *Natal measures* are of utmost importance, as mostly infection occurs during child birth. Deliveries should be conducted under hygienic conditions taking all aseptic measures. The new born baby's closed lids should be thoroughly cleansed and dried.
3. *Postnatal measures* include use of either ! percent tetracycline eye ointment or 0.5 percent erythromycin eye ointment. Crede's method

(not in use now) comprises use of 1% silver nitrate solution into the eyes of the babies immediately after birth.

Curative treatment

1. *Gonococcal ophthalmia neonatorum* is a serious condition and should be treated by following measures.
2. *Other bacterial ophthalmia neonatorum* should be treated by wide spectrum antibiotic drops and eye ointments.
3. *Neonatal inclusion conjunctivitis* responds well to topical tetracycline 1 percent eye ointment QID for 3 weeks.

VIRAL CONJUNCTIVITIS

Acute viral conjunctivitis may present in three clinical forms. Acute serous conjunctivitis, acute haemorrhagic conjunctivitis and acute follicular conjunctivitis.

Acute serous conjunctivitis

It is caused by mild grade viral infection which does not give rise to follicular response. It is characterized by a minimal congestion, a watery discharge and boggy swelling of the conjunctiva. Usually it is self-limiting and does not need any treatment.

Acute follicular conjunctivitis

It is an acute catarrhal conjunctivitis associated with marked follicular hyperplasia especially of the lower fornix and lower palpebral conjunctiva. Following types of acute follicular conjunctivitis caused by viruses are known :

1. *Epidemic keratoconjunctivitis.* It is mostly caused by adenoviruses type 8 and 19.
2. *Pharyngoconjunctival fever.* It is characteri-zed by an acute follicular conjunctivitis, associated with pharyngitis, fever and preauricular lymphadenopathy. It is commonly caused by adenovirus subtypes 3 and 7.
3. *Newcastle conjunctivitis* is a rare condition caused by New castle virus.
4. *Acute herpetic conjunctivitis* usually occur as a part of primary infection caused by herpes simplex virus type-I. It mainly occurs is small children and adolescents.

ADULT INCLUSION CONJUNCTIVITIS

It is a type of acute follicular conjunctivitis associated with mucopurolent discharge. It usually affects the sexually active young adults. It is caused by serotypes D to K of chlamydia trachomatis. The primary source of infection is urethritis in males and cervicitis in females. The transmission of infection may occur to eyes either through contaminated fingers or through contaminated water of swimming pools (hence the name *swimming pool conjunctivitis.*

TRACHOMA

Trachoma is a specific type of chronic conjunctivitis caused by chlamydia trachomatis. Its occurence is associated with poor socioeconomic status, poor sanitation and hygiene, dry and dusty weather; Infected finger, flies and fomites (use of common towel, handkerchief, bedding and surma-rods) play major role in its spread.

Prevalence. Trachoma is a worldwide disease but it is highly prevalent in North Africa, Middle East and certain regions of south east Asia (India, Iran China, Japan).

Clinical features

Symptoms. In the absence of secondary infection, symptoms are minimal and include mild foreign body sensation in the eyes, occasional lacrimation, slight stickiness of the lids and scanty mucoid discharge. In the presence of secondary infection typical symptoms of acute mucopurulent conjunctivitis develop.

Signs (Fig. 5.2)

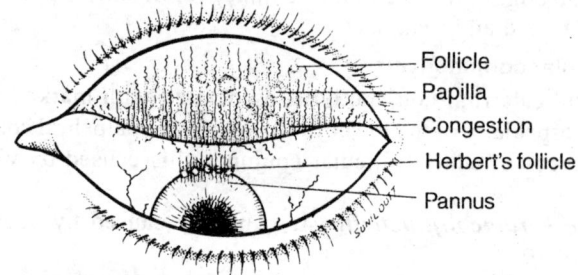

Follicle
Papilla
Congestion
Herbert's follicle
Pannus

Fig. 5.2. Signs of active trachoma.

1. *Conjunctival signs*
   - *Congestion* of upper tarsal and superior fornix conjunctiva.
   - *Follicles* look like boiled sago grains and are commonly seen on upper tarsal conjunctiva and superior fornix, but may also be present in the lower fornix, plica semilunaris and bulbar conjunctiva (pathognomic of trachoma).
   - *Papillae* are reddish flat-topped raised areas which give red and velvety appearance to the upper tarsal conjunctiva.
   - *Scarring* which may be irregular, star-shaped or linear is seen on the upper tarsal conjunctiva.

2. *Corneal signs*
   - *Superficial keratitis* may be present in the upper part.

- *Herbert's follicles* are present in the limbal area.
- *Pannus* refers to lymphoid infiltration with vascularization seen in the upper part of cornea.
- *Herbert's pits* are small circular pitted scars seen on the limbus.
- *Corneal opacity* may be present in the upper part which may extend down up to pupillary area.

WHO Classification

1. *Trachomatous inflammation follicular* (TF). It is characterized by presence of at least five or more follicles on the upper tarsal conjunctiva (Pl I.3).
2. *Trachomatous inflammation intense* (T.I). This stage is diagnosed when pronounced inflammatory thickening of the upper tarsal conjunctiva observer more than half of the normal deep tarsal vessels (Pl I.4).
3. *Trachomatous scarring* (TS). In this stage easily visible white scars are present on the upper tarsal conjunctiva (Pl I.5).
4. *Trachomatous trichiasis* (TT) is labelled when at least are misdirected eyelash rubs the eyeball (Pl I.6).
5. *Corneal opacity* (CO). This stage is labelled when easily visible corneal opacity is present over the pupillary area.

Sequelae and complications

1. *Sequelae in the lids* may be trichiasis, entropion, tylosis, ptosis.
2. *Conjunctival sequelae* include concretions, pseudocyst, xerosis and symblepharon.
3. *Corneal sequelae* include corneal xerosis and corneal opacity. Corneal ulcer may occur as a complication of misdirected cilia.

Diagnosis

1. *Clinical diagnosis* is made from by the presence of any two sets of signs out of the following :
   - Conjunctival follicles and papillae.
   - Pannus – progressive or regressive.
   - Epithelial keratitis near the superior limbus.
   - Star-shaped scarring of the upper tarsal conjunctiva.
2. *Laboratory diagnostic* tests employed for research purpose are as follows :
   - *Demonstration of inclusion bodies* in the conjunctival smear.
   - *Isolation of chlamydia* by yolk-sac inoculation method and tissue culture technique.
   - *Serotyping of TRIC agents* by micro-immunofluorescence method.

Treatment

An individual case of active trachoma may be treated by any of the following topical and systemic therapy regimes.

1. *Topical therapy regime.* It consists of 1% tetracycline or 1% erythromycin eye ointment 4 times a day for 6 weeks or 20% sulfacetamide eye drops three times a day along with 1% tetracyline eye ointment at bed time for 6 weeks.
2. *Systemic therapy regime* chosen may be any one of the following :
   - Tetracycline or Erythromycin 250 mg orally, four times a day for 3-4 weeks.
   - Doxycycline 100 mg orally twice daily for 3-4 weeks.
   - Single dose of Azathromycin 20 mg/kg body weight.
3. *Combined topical and systemic therapy* regime is preferred when the ocular infection is very severe or there is associated genital infection.

Prophylaxis

An ophthalmic nurse can play an important role in the prevention of trachoma and so should be well versed with the following prophylactic measures :

1. *Hygienic measures.* Health education on ocular hygiene is very useful. The use of common towel, handkerchief, surma rods etc should be discouraged. A good environmental sanitation will reduce the flies. A good water supply would improve washing habits.
2. *Early treatment of every case of conjunctivitis* helps in reducing the transmission of trachoma.
3. *WHO recommended blanket antibiotic* therapy regime for prevention. It includes use of 1% tetracycline eye ointment twice daily for 5 days in a month for 6 months.

ALLERGIC CONJUNCTIVITIS

It is the inflammation of conjunctiva due to allergic or hypersensitivity reactions. Conjunctiva is ten times more sensitive than skin to allergens. Common types of allergic conjunctivitis are as follows :

1. Simple allergic conjunctivitis
2. Vernal keratoconjunctivitis or spring catarrh.
3. Phlyctenular conjunctivitis.

SIMPLE ALLERGIC CONJUNCTIVITIS

Etiology. Simple allergic conjunctivitis is seen usually in the spring and summer and may result from exposure to allergens such as pollens and grass (seasonal allergic conjunctiva). Rarely it may also occur as an allergic response to perennial allergens such as house dust, mite and animal dandruff (Perennial allergic conjunctivitis).

Clinical features. It is a mild, non-specific, acute or subacute catarrhal conjunctivitis characterised by itching and discomfort in the eye; conjunctival hyperaemia and mild papillary hyperplasia.

Treatment
- *Non-steroidal antiallergic* eye drops 4-6 times a day.
- *Vasoconstrictor* such as naphazoline may also be useful.
- *Sodium chromoglycate* eye drops are useful in atopic cases.
- Steroid eye drops may be needed for short duration in severe and non-responsive cases.

VERNAL KERATOCONJUNCTIVITIS OR SPRING CATARRH. It is a specific type of allergic conjunctivitis characterized by recurrent, bilateral, self-limiting inflammation of the conjunctiva having a periodic seasonal incidence.

Etiology
It is due to hypersensitivity reaction to exogenous allergens such as grass pollens. It is mediated by IgE and may be associated with hay fever asthma or eczema.

Predisposing factors are as follows :
- *Age and sex.* 4-20 years, more common in boys than girls.
- *Season.* More common in summer.
- *Climate.* More prevalent in tropics, less in temperate zones and almost non-existent in cold climates.

Clinical features
Symptoms. Spring catarrh is characterized by marked *burning and itching sensation* which is usually intolerable and accentuated in warm humid atmosphere. *Ropy discharge* is characteristic. Other symptoms include mild photophobia, lacrimation and heaviness of lids.

Signs (Fig. 5.3). On the basis of signs spring catarrh can be divided into three clinical types :
1. *Palpebral form* is characterized by large papillae arranged in a 'cobble-stone' fashion on the upper tarsal conjunctiva of both eye (Pl. II.1). —
2. *Bulbar form* is characterized by dusky red triangular congestion of bulbar conjunctiva and gelatinous thickening of the upper limbal conjunctiva. discrete whitish dots (Tranta's spots) may also be present on the upper limbus.
3. *Mixed form* shows combined features of both palpebral and bulbar form.

Vernal keratopathy. Corneal involvement is associated with marked photophobia.

Treatment
1. *Steroid eye drops* should be used frequently for a short period only.
2. *Non-steroidal antiinflammatory* eye drops such as ketorolac may be used for a long period.
3. *Sodium cromoglycate (2%)* eye drops may be used four times a day. It stabilizes mast cells and thus prevents histamine release.
4. *Acetyl cysteine* 10-20% eye drops controls excess mucus formation.

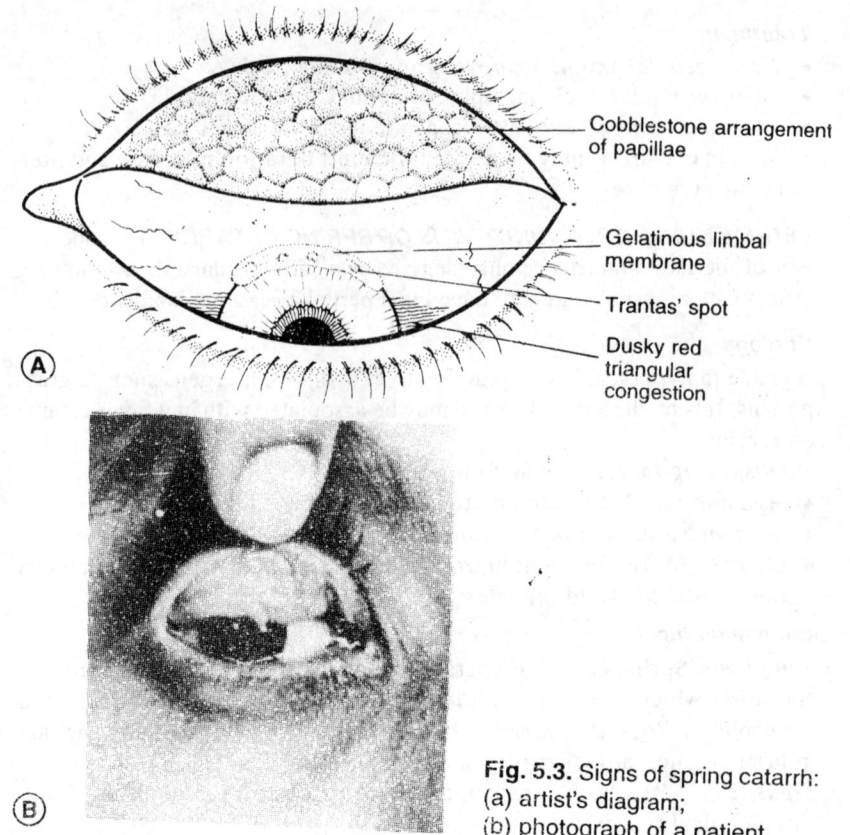

Cobblestone arrangement of papillae

Gelatinous limbal membrane

Trantas' spot

Dusky red triangular congestion

(A)

(B)

Fig. 5.3. Signs of spring catarrh:
(a) artist's diagram;
(b) photograph of a patient.

PHLYCTENULAR CONJUNCTIVITIS

It is a characteristic nodular affection of the conjunctiva occuring as an allergic response to some endogenous allergen.

Etiology. It is believed to be a delayed hypersensitivity (type IV-cell mediated) response to endogenous microbial proteins associated with:

• Tubercular infections in the body
• Staphylococcal infections such as tonsillitis and adenoids.
• Parasitic (worm) infestations.

Clinical features. Phlyctenular conjunctivitis is characterized by the presence of a typical pinkish white nodule surrounded by hyperaemia on the bulbar conjunctiva, usually near the limbus (Fig.5.4). Usually there is one nodule but may be more. Patients have symptoms like mild discomfort in the eye, irritation and watering. However, marked symptoms may be there due to associated mucopurulent conjunctivitis occuring as secondary infection. There may be associated phlyctenular keratitis.

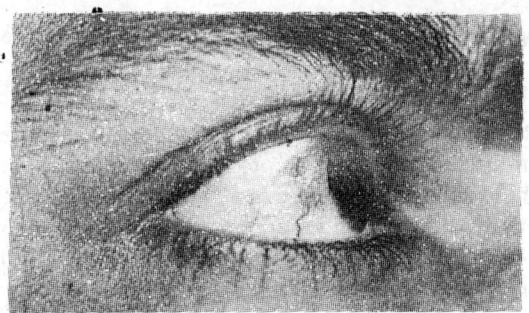

Fig. 5.4. Phylctenular conjunctivitis.

Treatment. It consists of topical șteroid and antibiotic drops. Attempts should be made to investigate the causative conditions and when discovered should be eradicated.

DEGENERATIVE CONDITIONS OF CONJUNCTIVA

PINGUECULA

Pinguecula is an extremely common degenerative condition of the conjunctiva. It is characterized by formation of a yellowish white patch on the bulbar conjunctiva near the limbus. It has been considered as an age-change, occurring moré commonly in persons exposed to strong sunlight, dust and wind. In routine no treatment is required for pinguecula as it is a symptomless condition.

PTERYGIUM

Pterygium (Fig.Pl II.2) is a wing shaped fold of conjunctiva encroaching upon the cornea. It occurs in the interpalpebral area more common on nasal than temporal side. *Etiology* is not known definitely. It is more common in people living in hot climates. Therefore, the most accepted view is that it is a response to prolonged effect of environmental factors such as exposure to sun (ultraviolet rays), dry heat,high wind and abundance of dust. *Surgical excision* is the only satisfactory treatment. However, recurrence is common after surgical treatment, which can be reduced by use of antimitotic drug and use of mucous membrane grafts.

CONCRETIONS

Concretions are yellowish white, hard looking, raised areas formed due to accumulation of inspissated mucous and dead epithelial cell debris into the crypts of palpebral conjunctiva. They usually remain as harmless spots but may cause irritation if they project beyond the surface, when they can be easily removed with the help of a hypodermic needle under topical anaesthesia.

SYMPTOMATIC CONDITIONS OF CONJUNCTIVA

SUBCONJUNCTIVAL HAEMORRHAGE

Subconjunctival haemorrhage is of very common occurrence. It may vary in extent from small petechial haemorrhage to an extensive area spreading under the whole of bulbar conjuctiva.

Etiology. It may occur after a severe bout of coughing or sneezing or, in the elderly, may be due to degenerative fragility of the capillaries. Other causes of subconjunctival haemorrhage include direct trauma, local vascular anomalies, blood dyscrasias and bleeding disorders.

Clinical features. Subconjunctival haemorrhage is a symptomless condition. It appears as a flat sheet of homogenous bright red colour with well defined margins. Most of the times it is absorbed completely within 7 to 21 days.

Treatment is not required usually except to reassure the patient that the redness will disappear. Treat the cause when discovered.

TUMOURS AND CYSTS OF CONJUNCTIVA

A staff nurse must, at least, be familiar with the names of various tumours and cysts of the conjunctiva. These are as follows ·

Tumours of conjunctiva

I. *Non-pigmented tumour*

1. *Congenital* : dermoid and lipodermoid.
2. *Benign :* simple granuloma, papilloma, adenoma, fibroma and angioma.
3. *Premalignant :* intraepithelial epithelioma (Bowen's disease).
4. *Malignant* : epithelioma or squamous cell carcinoma, basal cell carcinoma.

II. *Pigmented tumours*

1. *Benign :* naevi or congenital moles.
2. *Precancerous melanosis* : superficial spreading melanoma.
3. *Malignant :* melanoma

Cysts of the conjunctiva

1. Congenital : epibulbar dermoid
2. Lymphatic cyst
3. Retention cyst.
4. Epithelial implantation cyst.
5. Aqueous cyst
6. Parasitic cyst e.g. subconjunctival cysticercus.

6

Diseases of Cornea and Sclera

DISEASES OF CORNEA

The cornea is a transparent, avascular, watch glass-like structure. It forms the anterior one-sixth of the outer fibrous coat of the eyeball. The exposed position of cornea is the principal reason why it is vulnerable to pathology by accidental trauma and ulceration. The common disorders of cornea include its inflammations (keratitis), traumatic lacerations, degenerations and dystrophies, ultimately leading to corneal opacification and to marked loss of vision.

KERATITIS

Inflammation of the cornea, keratitis, is a common condition. It is characterized by corneal oedema, cellular infilteration and ciliary congestion.

Classifications

Topographical (morphological) classification
1. *Ulcerative keratitis (corneal ulcer)*
   - Purulent corneal ulcer
   - Nonpurulent corneal ulcer
2. *Nonulcerative keratitis*
   - Superficial keratitis
   - Deep keratitis
     - Interstitial keratitis
     - Disciform keratitis

Etiological classification
1. *Infective keratitis,* which depending upon the causative organism may be bacterial, viral, fungal, chlamydial, protozoal or spirochaetal.
2. *Allergic keratitis* includes phlyctenular keratitis, vernal keratopathy and atopic keratitis.

3. *Trophic keratitis* includes exposure keratitis and neurotrophic keratitis.
4. *Traumatic keratitis* which may be due to mechanical trauma, chemical burns or thermal burns.
5. *Idiopothic keratitis,* e.g. Mooren's corneal ulcer.

ULCERATIVE KERATITIS

Ulcerative keratitis, also known as corneal ulcer, is the inflammation of cornea associated with some destruction of a portion of epithelium. It may be purulent or non-purulent. Most of the bacterial and fungal corneal ulcers are purulent (suppurative) while most of the viral, chlamydial and allergic corneal ulcers are non-purulent.Some of the common varieties of corneal ulcers are dealt with.

Bacterial corneal ulcer

Etiology

Common bacteria associated with corneal ulceration are *Staphylococcus aureus, Pseudomonas pyocyanea, Streptococcus pneumoniae, E. coli, Proteus, Klebsiella, N. gonorrhoea, N. menignitidis* and *C. diphtheriae. Prerequisites* for most of the bacteria to produce corneal ulceration is corneal epithelial damage, except the last three which can invade the intact corneal epithelium.

Clinical features

Symptoms

1. *Photophobia* i.e. intolerance to light is the most characteristic symptom of keratitis.
2. *Pain* occurs due to irritation of the exposed nerve endings.
3. *Watering and redness* of eyes are also present.
4. *Defective vision* occurs due to corneal haze.

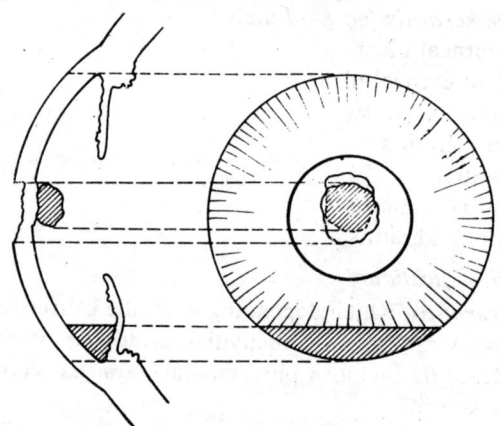

Fig. 6.1. Hypopyon corneal ulcer.

Signs

1. *Lids* are swollen.
2. *Blepharospasm* is usually marked.
3. *Conjunctiva* is chemosed and hyperaemic.
4. *Cornea* shows ulcer in the form of a yellowish white pit on the surface; which can be readily demonstrated after instillation of a drop of 2% freshly prepared solution of fluorescein dye. The ulcerated area being denuded of epithelium stains green.
5. *Anterior chamber* may or may not show pus (hypopyon) (Pl II.3). Development of hypopyon depends upon the virulence of organism and resitance of the patient. The characteristic hypopyon ulcer caused by pneumococcus is called *ulcus serpens* (Fig. 6.1).

Treatment

1. *Topical antibiotics* as eye drops should be used very frequently in the day and as eye ointment at night.
2. *Topical cycloplegic drugs,* preferably 1% atropine eye ointment or eye drops should be used to reduce pain from ciliary spasm and to give rest to the eye.
3. *Systemic analgesics* may be required to relieve pain.
4. *Vitamins* like A, B-complex and C, may help in early healing of the ulcer.
5. *Hot fomentation* gives comfort, reduces pain and causes vasodilatation.

Fungal corneal ulcer

The incidence of suppurative corneal ulcers caused by fungi has increased in the recent years due to injudicious use of antibiotics and steroids.

Etiology

Common causative fungi are *Aspergillus, Candida* and *Fusarium*.
Mode of infection is usually a trauma by vegetative material such as crop leaf, branch of a tree, straw, hay or decaying vegetable matter.

Clinical features

Symptoms are similar to bacterial corneal ulcer except that comparatively they are less marked than the signs.
Signs, in general, are also similar to suppurative bacterial corneal ulcer. A *typical fungal corneal ulcer* is dry looking having thick greyish white slough at the base. Multiple small satellite lesions may be present around the ulcer. Usually a big hypopyon is present even if the ulcer is very small.

Diagnosis

Clinical diagnosis may be supplemented by laboratory investigations which include examination of wet KOH, Gram's and Giemsa stained films for fungal hyphae and culture on Sabouraud's agar medium.

Treatment

Specific treatment consists of *antifungal drugs* such as natamycin, fluconazole, nystatin and silver sulfadiazine in the form of frequently instilled eye drops. Other measures are similar to bacterial corneal ulcer.

Viral corneal ulcers

Common viral infections include herpes simplex keratitis, herpes zoster ophthalmicus and adenovirus keratitis.

Herpes simplex keratitis

Ocular infection with herpes simplex virus (HSV) are extremely common. Herpes simplex virus, a DNA virus is of two types – type-I typically causes infection above the waist and type-II below the waist (herpes genitalis).

Mode of infection

HSV-I infection is primarily acquired by kissing or coming in close contact with a patient suffering from herpes labialis.

HSV-II infection is transmitted to eyes of neonates through infected genitalia of the mother.

Ocular lesions of herpes simplex

Ocular involvement by HSV occurs in two forms : primary and recurrent.

Primary ocular herpes infection (first attack) involves a non-immune person. It typically occurs in children between 6 months and 5 years of age and also in teenagers. Its features are :

1. *Vesicular skin lesions* may involve lids and periorbital region.
2. *Acute follicular conjunctivitis* is the usual and sometimes the only manifestation.
3. *Epithelial keratitis* occurs in less than half of the cases.

   Primary infection is usually self- limiting but the virus travels up to trigeminal ganglion and establishes the latent infection.

Recurrent ocular herpes infection occurs due to periodic reactivation of the virus lying dormant in the trigeminal ganglion. *Predisposing stress stimuli* which trigger an attack of herpetic keratitis include fever such as malaria, flu, exposure to ultraviolet rays, general ill health, emotional or physical exhaustion and mild trauma. Its features are :

1. *Epithelial keratitis* initially occurs as fine or coarse superficial punctate keratitis (Fig. 6.2A). The typical lesion of recurrent epithelial keratitis is *dendritic ulcer,* a zig-zag linear branching ulcer (Fig 6.2 B and Pl II.4). Sometimes the branches of dendritic ulcer enlarge and coalesce to form a large ulcer with a *geographical or amoeboid* configuration (Fig. 6.2 C). Symptoms of epithelial keratitis are pain, photophobia, lacrimation and blurred vision.

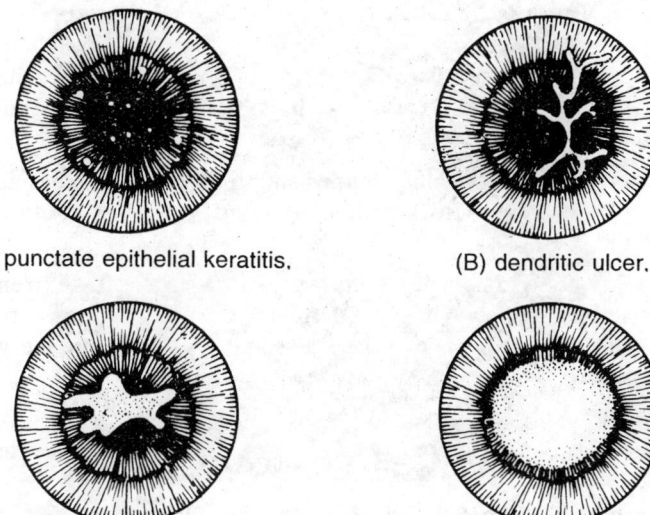

(A) punctate epithelial keratitis.   (B) dendritic ulcer.

(C) geographical ulcer   (D) disciform keratitis.

Fig. 6.2. Lesions of recurrent herpes simplex keratitis:

Specific treatment consists of frequent use of antiviral drops such as 0.1 per cent idoxuridine (IDU) drops or 3% acyclovir ointment.

2. *Stromal keratitis* in the form of *disciform keratitis* (Fig. 6.2D) may occur due to delayed hypersensitivity reaction to HSV antigen.

  Its treatment consists of diluted steroid eye drops instilled 4-5 times a day with an antiviral cover (acyclovir 3% twice a day).

Herpes zoster ophthalmicus

Herpes zoster ophthalmicus is an acute infection of gasserian ganglion of the fifth cranial nerve by the varicella-zoster virus (VZV).

Etiology

The infection is contracted in childhood, which manifests as chickenpox. The virus then remains dormant in the trigeminal ganglion and reactivates later, when the immunity is depressed to cause herpes zoster.

Clinical features

General features include fever, malaise and severe neuralgic pain along the course of the affected nerve.

Cutaneous lesions (Fig.6.3) include vesicles in the area of distribution of the involved nerve which may be converted into pustules and ultimately heal by pitted scars.

Ocular lesions appear in about 50 per cent cases of herper zoster

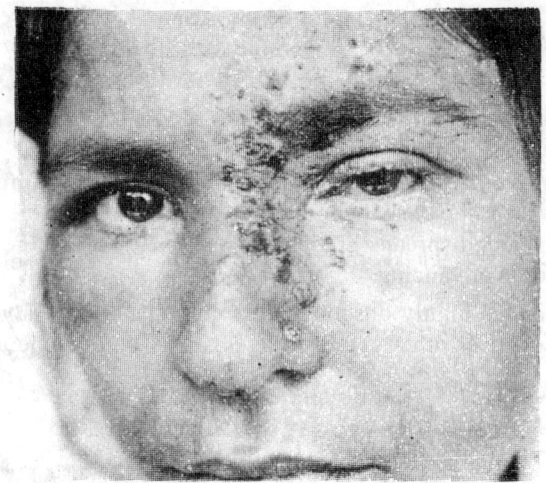

Fig. 6.3. Cutaneous lesions of herpes zoster ophthalmicus.

ophthalmicus and may be in the form of conjunctivitis, keratitis, episcleritis and iridocyclitis. Zoster keratitis may occur as fine or coarse epithelial keratitis, nummular keratitis or disciform keratitis.

Treatment

1. *Analgesics* for severe pain
2. *Systemic acyclovir* 800 mg 5 times a day for 10 days.
3. *Antibiotic steroid* ointment for scar lesions.
4. *Systemic steroids* may be required if other cranial nerves are also involved.
5. *Zoster keratitis* should be treated by topical acyclovir eye ointment, cyclopentolate and steroid drops.

Exposure keratitis

Etiology. Exposure keratitis develops when the eyeball is insufficiently covered by the lids and there is loss of protective mechanism of blinking. It may occur in patients with :

1. Extreme proptosis
2. Facial nerve palsy
3. Severe ectropion
4. Inadequate closure of lids in deep coma.

Clinical features. Initial dessication occurs in the interpalpebral area leading to fine or punctate keratitis which is followed by necrosis, frank ulceration and vascularization.

Treatment. Artificial tears and ointment should be applied frequently. Cornea should be kept covered and the causative condition should be treated. Tarsorrhaphy should be performed when the treatment of cause is not possible.

Mooren's ulcer

Mooren's ulcer is a severe inflammatory peripheral ulcerative keratitis of unknown etiology.

Clinical features. Mooren's ulcer is a chronic, very painful, indolent ulcer usually seen in elderly people. The ulcer begins near the upper margin of the cornea and spreads gradually; whilst one part of the ulcer is healing the other is advancing.

Treatment is highly unsatisfactory. Immuno-suppressive drugs such as *cyclosporine* or other cytotoxic agents may be of some use.

NON-ULCERATIVE KERATITIS

Interstitial keratitis

Interstitial keratitis denotes an inflammation of the corneal stroma without ulceration.

Etiology. Common causes of interstitial keratitis are congenital syphilis, tuberculosis, acquired syphilis and lerprosy.

Clinical features. The condition is characterized by marked oedema of the corneal stroma, giving a ground glass appearance, with associated signs of anterior uveitis. Deep vascularization of cornea may occur in florid stage of inflammation. Usually, there occurs a severe loss of vision.

Treatment consists of systemic treatment for the underlying cause and topical steroids and cycloplegics for controlling the corneal inflammation. Keratoplasty may be required where dense corneal opacities are left.

CORNEAL DEGENERATIONS AND DYSTROPHIES

CORNEAL DEGENERATIONS

Arcus senilis

Arcus senilis refers to an annular infilteration of corneal periphery. It is a symptomless age-related degeneration occuring bilaterally in old persons. It does not affect the vision or vitality of cornea and so requires no treatment.

Fatty degeneration of cornea

Fatty degeneration of cornea, also known as lipoid keratopathy, is characterized by yellowish white deposits in the cornea. It usually occurs secondary to corneal vascularization associated with long standing keratitis, corneal injuries and chronic corneal oedema due to any cause.

Band-shaped keratopathy

Band-shaped keratopathy, also known as calcific degeneration of cornea, is essentially a degenerative change associated with deposition of calcium salts in Bowman's membrane, most superficial parts of the stroma and in deeper layers of epithelium.

Causes. It may occur rarely as a primary condition associated with hypercalcemia. Usually it occurs as a secondary condition associated with chronic uveitis in adults, Still's disease in children, phthisis bulbi, absolute glaucoma.

Clinical features. It typically presents as a band shaped opacity in the interpalpebral zone with a clear interval between the ends of the band and limbus.

Treatment. (1) *Chemical removal of deposited calcium salts* with a chelating agent (EDTA) may be useful. (2) *Phototherapeutic keratectomy (PTK)* with excimer laser is very effective in clearing the cornea. (3) *Keratoplasty* may be considered when band- shaped keratopathy is obscuring the useful vision.

CORNEAL DYSTROPHIES

Corneal dystrophies are inhereted disorders characterized by development of corneal haze in otherwise normal eyes that are free from inflammation or vascularization. There is no associated systemic disease. Dystrophies occur bilaterally, manifesting occasionally at birth, but more usually during first or second decade and sometimes even later in life.

Classification. Corneal dystrophies may be classified as below :

1. *Anterior dystrophies.* These primarily affect epithelium and Bowman's layer.
2. *Stromal dystrophies.* These primarily involve corneal stroma and include granular dystrophy, lattice dystrophy and macular dytrophy.
3. *Posterior dystrophies.* These primarily involve the corneal endothelium and Descemet's membrane. Examples of posterior dytrophies are corneal guttata and Fuch's epithelial-endothelial dystrophy.
4. *Ectatic dystrophies* include keratoconus and keratoglobus.

Keratoconus

Keratoconus (conical cornea) is a non-inflammatory, bilateral (85%), ectatic condition of cornea involving its axial part (Fig.6.4). It usually starts at puberty and progresses slowly.

Clinical features. Patient presents with a defective vision due to progressive myopia with irregular astigmatism which does not improve despite full correction with glasses.

Signs of keratoconus are as follows :

- Conical shape of the cornea
- Window reflex is distorted
- Placido disc examination shows irregularity of the circles.
- Slit lamp examination may show thinning and ectasia of central cornea fine opacity at the apex and Fleischer's ring at the base of cone.

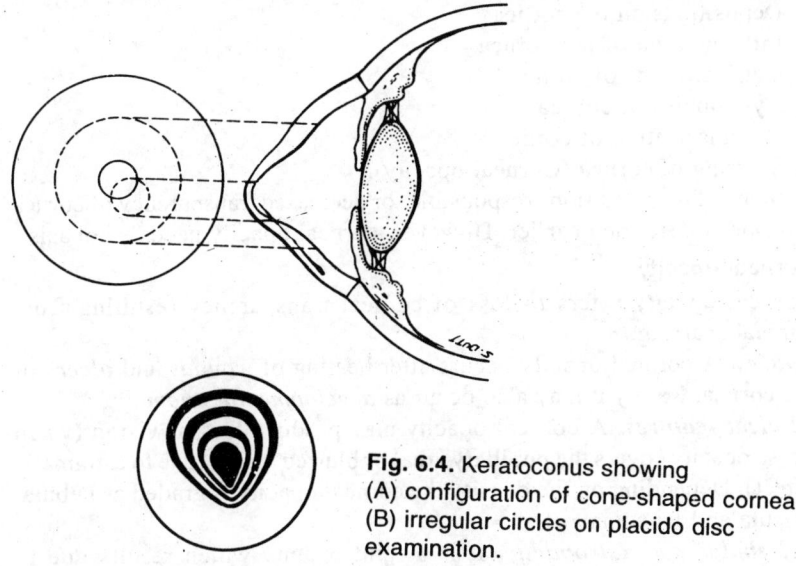

Fig. 6.4. Keratoconus showing
(A) configuration of cone-shaped cornea;
(B) irregular circles on placido disc
examination.

- On retinoscopy a yawning reflex and high oblique or irregular astigmatism is obtained.
- On distant direct ophthalmoscopy a dark ring reflex in seen due to total internal reflection of light.
- Munson's sign, i.e. localized indentation of the lower lid while looking down is positive in late stages.

Treatment. Spectacles are usually not helpful. *Hard contact lenses* are useful in early cases. *Penetrating keratoplasty* may be required in advanced cases.

Keratoglobus

It is a familial and hereditary, bilateral congenital disorder characterized by thinning and hemispherical protrusion of the entire cornea. It is non-progressive and inherited as an autosomal recessive trait. It must be differentiated from buphthalmos in which enlarged cornea is associated with raised intraocular pressure, anomalies of the angle of anterior chamber and cupping of the optic disc.

ABNORMALITIES OF CORNEAL TRANSPARENCY

Normal cornea is a transparent structure. Almost any process which upsets its anatomy or physiology causes loss of its transparency to some degree.
Common causes of loss of corneal transparency are :
- Corneal oedema
- Drying of cornea

- Depositions on the cornea
- Inflammation of the cornea
- Degenerations of cornea
- Dystrophies of cornea
- Vascularization of cornea
- Scarring of cornea (Corneal opacity).

Some of the conditions responsible for decreased transparency of cornea have been described earlier. However, corneal opacity needs emphasis.

Corneal opacity

Corneal opacity refers to loss of corneal transparency resulting from corneal scarring.

Causes. A corneal opacity occurs after healing of *wounds* and *ulcers* of the cornea. Rarely it may also occur as *developmental anomaly.*

Clinical features. A corneal opacity may produce loss of vision (when dense opacity covers the pupillary area) or blurred vision (due to astigmatic effect). Depending on the density the corneal opacity is graded as nebula, macula and leucoma.

1. *Nebular corneal opacity.* It is a faint opacity which results due to superficial scar involving Bowman's layer and superficial stroma (Fig.6.5A). Details of the iris are visible through this faint opacity.

2. *Macular corneal opacity.* It is a semidense whitish opacity produced when scarring involves about half of the corneal stroma (Fig.6.5 B).

3. *Leucomatous corneal opacity (leucoma simplex).* It is a thick, dense white opacity which results when almost full thickness of cornea is involved (Fig.6.5 C).

4. *Adherent leucoma* results when healing occurs after perforation of cornea with incarceration of iris (Fig.6.5 D and Fig. 6.6).

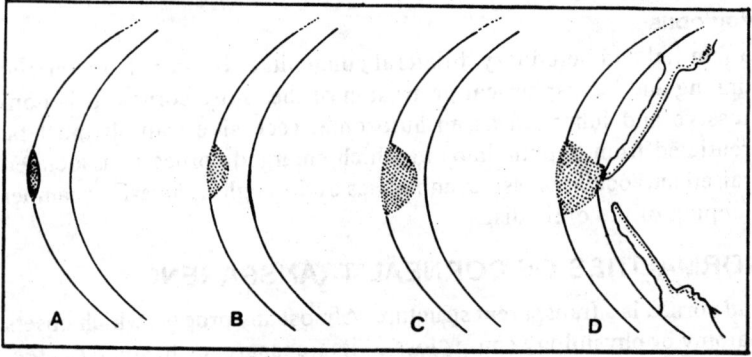

Fig. 6.5. Corneal opacity:
(A) nebular; (B) macular; (C) leucomatous; (D) adherent leucoma.

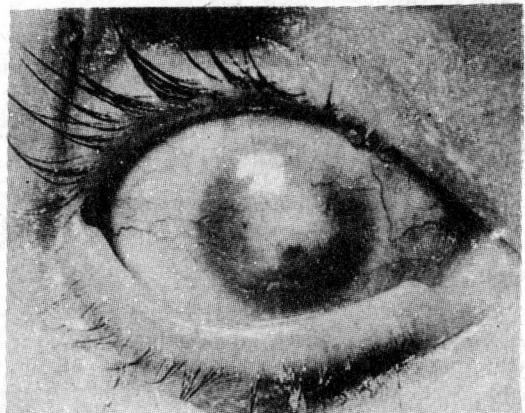

Fig. 6.6. Vascularised adherent leucoma.

KERATOPLASTY

Keratoplasty, also called as corneal grafting or corneal transplantation,is an operation in which the patient's diseased cornea is replaced by the donor's healthy cornea.

Types

1. Penetrating keratoplasty (full thickness grafting).
2. Lamellar keratoplasty (partial thickness grafting).

Indications

1. *Optical*, i.e., to improve vision. Important indications are corneal opacity, bullous keratopathy, corneal dytrophies and advanced keratoconus.
2. *Therapeutic,* i.e. to replace inflamed cornea not responding to conventional therapy.
3. *Tectonic grafts*, i.e, to restore integrity of eyeball, e.g. after corneal perforation and marked corneal thining.
4. *Cosmetic* i.e., to improve the appearance of badly scarred eye.

Donor tissue. The donor eyes should be removed as early as possible, preferably within 6 hours of death of the donor. The donor eye to be useful must be free from corneal diseases. The eyes should be stored under sterile conditions.

Nurses may be asked by patients or their relatives how to donate their eyes to a bank after death. Some hospitals have a leaflet giving information on the subject. It will be best for a nurse to be familiar with all about eye donations.

Methods of corneal preservation

The eyes are prepared in various ways and the nurse will need to become familiar with the method in use in the hospital in which she is working. Common methods of storage are as below:

1. *Short-term storage* (upto 48 hours). The whole globe is preserved at 4°C in a moist chamber. The eyes to be used for a full- thickness graft must be used within 48 hours.

2. *Intermediate storage* (upto 2 weeks) of donor cornea can be done in McCarey-Kaufman (MK) medium and various chondroitin -sulfate enriched media such as optisol medium.

3. *Long-term storage* upto 35 days can be done by organ culture method.

Surgical technique

The keratoplasty operation can be described in three stages :

1. *Preparation of the donor material.* The donor corneal button should be prepared first and kept safely. It should be cut 0.25 mm larger than the recipient button taking care not to damage the endothelium. From the stored cornea, the button should be cut from endothelial side over a teflon block (Fig.6.7 A), alternatively, from the whole eyeball the donor button can be prepared by a technique similar to that of excision of recipient corneal button (Fig.6.7 B).

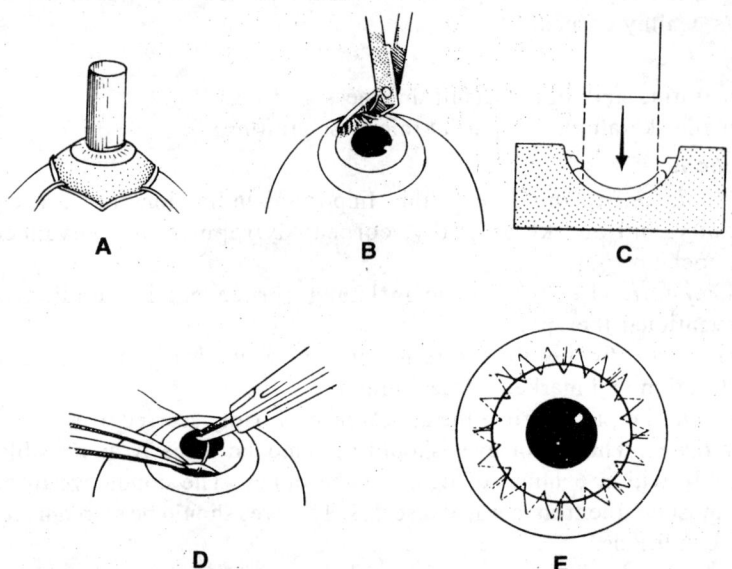

Fig. 6.7. Technique of keratoplasty: (A&B) excision of recipient corneal button; (C) excision of donor corneal button; (D) suturing of donor button into recipient's bed; (E) showing pattern of continuous sutures in keratoplasty.

2. *Excision of the recipient corneal button* with the help of a corneal trephine (7.5 mm to 8 mm in diameter) a partial thickness incision is made in the host cornea (Fig.6.7 B). Then the anterior chamber is entered with the half of a razor blade knife and excision is completed using corneo-scleral scissors (Fig. 6.7 C).

3. *Suturing of corneal graft into the host bed* (Fig. 6.7 D) is performed with either interrupted or continuous 10-0 nylon suture (Fig. 6.7 E and Pl II.5) .

A staff nurse should be familiar with the steps of the operation and also with all the instruments required for this operation.

Postoperative care

1. *General nursing care* for this patient is same as for the patient who has undergone a cataract operation (see page 41-44 and 139).

2. *Postoperative dressing* should be carried out daily for a week using antibiotic and steroid drops and ointment.

3. *Postoperative treatment* in the form of dark goggles, antibiotic and steroid eye drops need to be continued for 3-4 months.

4. *Suture removal if required* may be performed after 4 months.

DISEASES OF SCLERA

EPISCLERITIS

It is a benign, recurrent inflammation of the episcleral tissue involving the overlying Tenon's capsule. It typically affects young adults, being twice as common in women than men.

Etiology

Exact etiology is not known. It is found in association with gout, rosacea, rheumatoid arthritis and psoriasis. It has also been reported to occur as an allergic reaction to endogenous proteins or toxins.

Clinical features

Symptoms of episclerits include a localized redness and mild ocular discomfort.ı

Signs. In nodular episclerits a pink or purple flat nodule usually situated 2-3 mm away from the limbus is seen. The nodule is firm, tender and the overlying conjunctiva moves over it. In diffuse episcleritis inflammation involves one or two quadrants of the episcleral tissue.

Treatment

Treatment of episcleritis includes topical corticosteroid eye drops, systemic non-steroidal anti-inflammatory durgs (e.g. flurbiprofen) and cold compresses.

SCLERITIS

It is an inflammation of the scleral tissue (sclera proper). It usually occurs in elderly people (40-70 years) involving females more than males.

Etiology

It is found in association with multiple conditions which are as follows :

1. *Autoimmune collagen disorders* are associated in 50% cases, most common being rheumatoid arthritis. Other associated disorders are polyarteritis nodosa, systemic lupus erythematosus, Wegner's granulomatosis and dermatomyositis.
2. *Metabolic disorders* like gout and thyrotoxicosis may be associated with some cases.
3. *Infections,* particularly herpes zoster ophthalmicus and staphylococcus are known to cause scleritis.
4. *Granulomatous diseases* like tuberculosis, syphilis, sarcoidosis and leprosy can also cause scleritis.
5. *Idiopathic scleritis* occurs in many cases.

Classification

Scleritis can be classified as follows:

1. ***Anterior scleritis***
    1. *Non-necrotizing scleritis*
        (a) Diffuse
        (b) Nodular
    2. *Necrotizing scleritis*
        (a) with inflammation
        (b) without inflammation (scleromalacia perforans).

II. ***Posterior scleritis***

Clinical features

Symptoms. Patients complain of moderate to severe *pain* which is deep and boring in character. It s associated with localized or diffuse *redness,* mild to severe *photophobia* and *lacrimation.*

Signs. Salient features of different clinical varieties of scleritis are as follows :

1. *Non-necrotizing anterior diffuse scleritis.* It is characterized by widespread inflammation involving a quadrant or more of the anterior sclera. The involved area is raised and salmon pink to purple in colour.
2. *Non-necrotizing anterior nodular scleritis.* It is characterized by one or two hard, purplish, elevated scleral nodules, usually situated near the limbus (Pl II.6).
3. *Anterior necrotizing scleritis with inflammation.* It is an acute severe form of scleritis characterized by intense localized inflammation associated with areas of infarction due to vasculitis.

4. *Anterior necrotizing scleritis without inflammation. (Scleromalacia perforans).* It typically occurs in elderly females suffering from long standing rheumatoid arthritis and is characterized by a yellowish patch of melting sclera (due to obliteration of arterial supply).

5. *Posterior scleritis.* It refers to inflammation of sclera posterior to equator which is often complicated by exudative retinal detachment, macular oedema, proptosis and limitation of ocular movements.

Treatment

1. *Non-necrotizing scleritis* is treated by topical steroid eye drops and systemic indomethacin.

2. *Necrotizing scleritis* is treated by topical steroids and heavy doses of oral steroids, tapered slowly.

BLUE SCLERA

It is an asymptomatic condition characterized by marked, generalized blue discolouration due to thinning. It is a typical association of osteogenesis imperfecta.

STAPHYLOMAS

Staphyloma refers to localized bulging of weak and thin outer tunic of the eyeball (cornea or sclera), lined by uveal tissue which shines through the thinned-out fibrous coat.

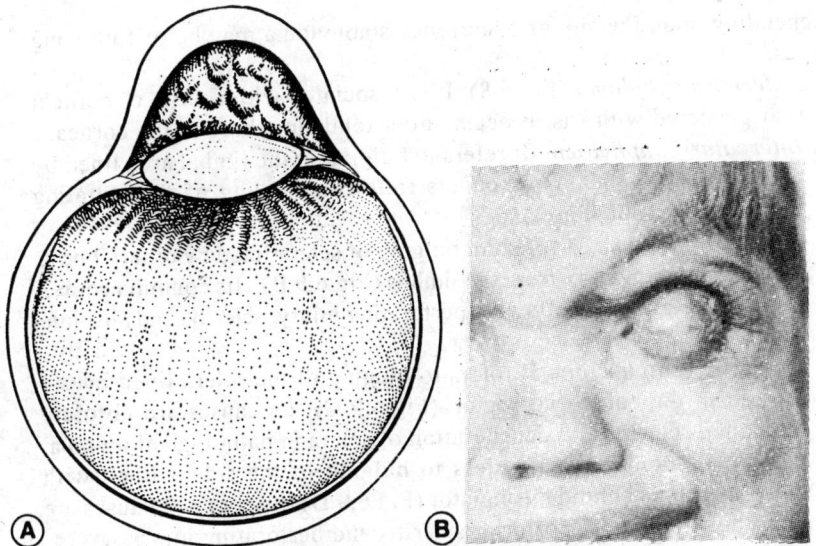

Fig. 6.8. Anterior staphyloma: (A) diagrammatic cross-section; (B) clinical photograph.

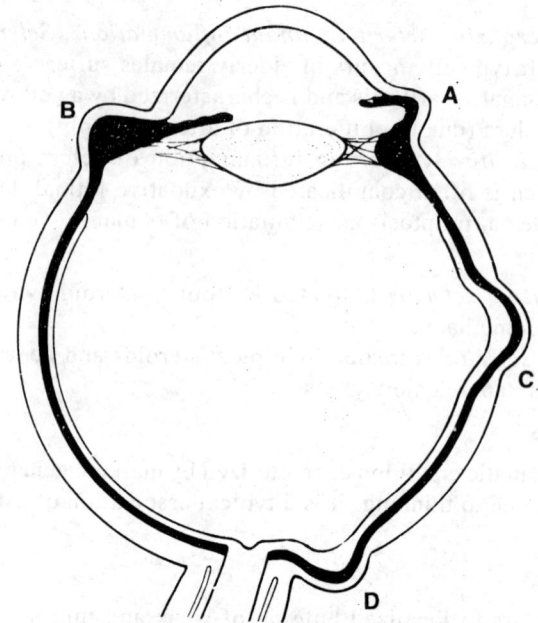

Fig. 6.9. Staphylomas: (A) intercalary; (B) ciliary;
(C) equatorial; (D) posterior.

Clinical types

Depending upon the site of occurrence staphyloma may be of following types:

1. *Anterior staphyloma* (Fig 6.8). It is associated with ectasia of corneal scar plastered with iris. It occurs after total sloughing of the cornea.
2. *Intercalary staphyloma.* It refers to bulging in the limbal area lined by coat of iris (Fig.6.9 A). It occurs following healing of a perforating injury in the limbal area.
3. *Ciliary staphyloma.* It refers to bulging of sclera lined by ciliary body. It occurs 2-3 mm away from the limbus (Fig.6.9 B). Its common causes are thinning of sclera following perforating injury, scleritis and absolute glaucoma.
4. *Equatorial staphyloma.* It refers to bulging of the sclera lined by the choroid in the equatorial region (Fig.6.9 C). Its causes are absolute glaucoma, scleritis and degeneration of sclera in pathological myopia.
5. *Posterior staphyloma.* It refers to bulging of the sclera lined with choroidal tissue behind the equator (Fig.6.9 D). Its common causes are pathological myopia, posterior scleritis and perforating injuries.

7

Diseases of the Uveal Tract

CONGENITAL ANOMALIES

1. Heterochromia of iris. It refers to variations in the iris colour. In *heterochromia iridum* colour of one iris differs from the other and in *heretrochomia iridis* colour of one sector of the iris differs from the rest of iris.

2. Polycoria. It refers to congenital presence of more than one pupil.

3. Congenital aniridia or iridremia. It refers to congenital absence of iris.

4. Persistent pupillary membrane. It represents the remnants of the anterior vascular sheath of the lens which normally disappears before birth. It is characterized by the stellate-shaped shreds of the pigmented tissue coming from the anterior surface of iris.

5. Coloboma of the uveal tract. Coloboma (absence of a part of tissue) of iris, ciliary body and choroid may be seen in association or independently.

UVEITIS

The term uveitis refers to inflammation of the uveal tract.

Classification

I. *Anatomical classification*

1. *Anterior uveitis* or iridocyctitis. It is the inflammation of iris and pars plicata part of the ciliary body.
2. *Intermediate uveitis* or pars planitis refers to the pars plana part of ciliary body.
3. *Posterior uveitis* or choroiditis is the inflammation of the choroid.
4. *Panuveitis* is inflammation of the whole uvea.

II. *Clinical classification*

1. *Acute uveitis*
2. *Chronic uveitis*

III. *Pathological classification*

i. *Suppurative or purulent uveitis*

    2. *Non-suppurative uveitis.*
      (i) Non-granulomatous uveitis
      (ii) Granulomatous uveitis
IV. *Etiological classification*
   See etiology

Etiology of Uveitis

Depending upon the etiology, uveitis can be classified as below :

1. *Infective uveitis* is induced by invasion of the tissue by micro-organisms. Uveal infections may be exogenous, secondary or endogenous. Depending upon the causative organism the infective uveitis may be bacterial, viral, fungal parasitic.
2. *Allergic uveitis.* It is of the commonest occurence in clinical practice. Allergy or hypersensitivity-linked uveitis may occur as uveitis due to microbial allergy, atopic uveitis, autoimmune uveitis or HLA-associated uveitis.
3. *Toxic uveitis.* It is caused by direct effects of some toxins on the uveal tissue. Toxins responsible for uveitis may be endotoxins, endocular toxins or endogenous toxins.
4. *Traumatic uveitis* may be associated with accidental or operative trauma.
5. *Uveitis associated with non-infective systemic diseases.* It occurs in patients with sarcoidosis, collagen disorders (rheumatoid arthritis, polyartritis nodosa) and metabolic disorders (diabetes mellitus and gout).
6. *Idiopathic uveitis.* In more than 25 percent of cases uveitis is of unknown etiology.

ANTERIOR UVEITIS (IRIDOCYCLITIS)

It refers to inflammation of the iris and ciliary body. Clinically, it may occur as acute or chronic iridocyclitis.

Clinical features

Symptoms

1. *Pain* in the eye radiating to other parts of the face is a dominating symptom of acute iridocyclitis. It is worse at night. In chronic uveitis pain may be minimal or absent.
2. *Redness* occurs due to congestion of circumcorneal vessels. In chronic iridocyclitis eye may be white.
3. *Photophobia and lacrimation* occurs due to irritation of the sensory nerves.
4. *Defective vision* may occur due to haze in the aqueous humour, exudates in the pupillary area and vitreous opacities.

Signs (Fig 7.1 and Pl III.1)

1. *Lid oedema,* usually mild may be present in a patient with severe attack of acute iridocyclitis.

2. *Circumcorneal congestion* is marked in acute iridocyclitis. It must be differentiated from the superficial congestion occuring in acute conjunctivitis (see table 5.1 , page 87). In chronic iridocyclitis congestion is minimum.

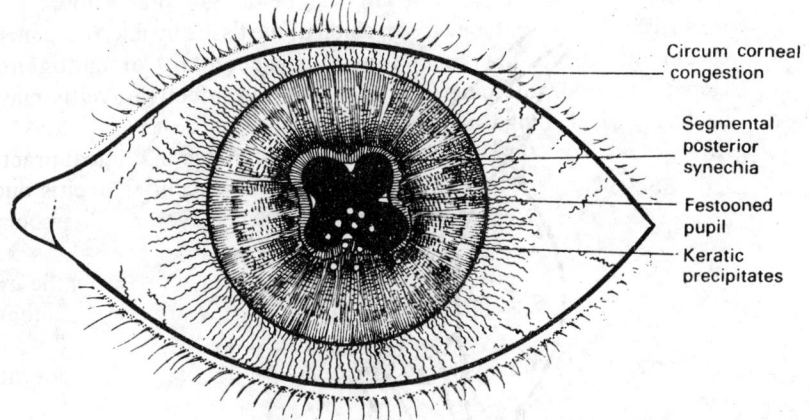

Circum corneal congestion

Segmental posterior synechia

Festooned pupil

Keratic precipitates

Fig. 7.1. Signs of anterior uveitis.

3. *Corneal signs*

   I. Corneal oedema is usually mild

   II. Keratic prcepitates (KPs) are proteinaceous cellular deposits occuring at the back of cornea (Fig.7.2). These may be small and medium (granular) KPs or large mutton-fat KPs. Fresh KPs are usually circular and grey-coloured while old KPs are small, pigmented and have crenated edges.

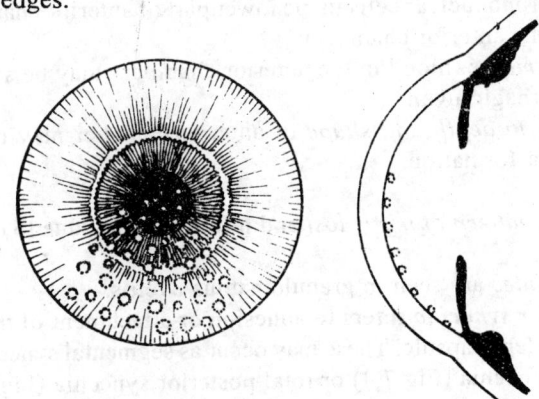

Fig. 7.2. Keratic precipitates (KPs).

4. Anterior chamber signs

i. *Aqueous cells.* Presence of inflammatory cells in the aqueous humour is a sign of active inflammation.

ii. *Aqueous flare.* It is due to leakage of proteins into the aqueous through the damaged capillaries. Aqueous flare is best demonstrated in the fine beam of a slit-lamp as suspended and moving dust particles (Fig.7.3).

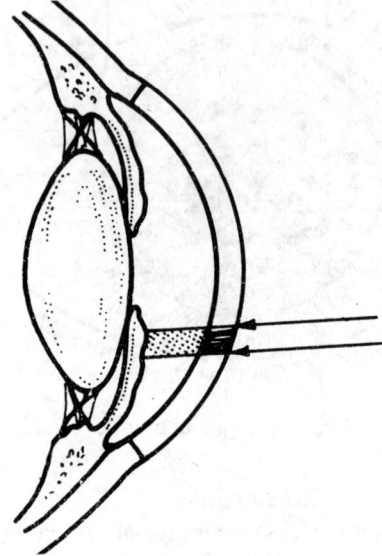

Fig. 7.3. Aqueous flare.

iii. *Hypopyon* occurs in severe cases due to collection of polymorphonuclear cells in the lower part of anterior chamber (sterile pus in the anterior chamber).

iv. *Hyphaema* i.e. blood in the anterior chamber may be seen rarely in haemorrhagic uveitis.

v. *Change in depth and shape* of anterior chamber may occur due to synechia formation.

5. Iris signs

i. Normal *pattern of iris is lost* and it looks muddy due to collection of exudates.

ii. *Iris nodules* are seen in granulomatous uveitis.

iii. *Posterior synechia* refers to adhesion or attachment of the iris to the anterior lens capsule. These may occur as segmental synechia, annular (ring) synechia (Fig 7.4) or total posterior synechia (Fig. 7.5).

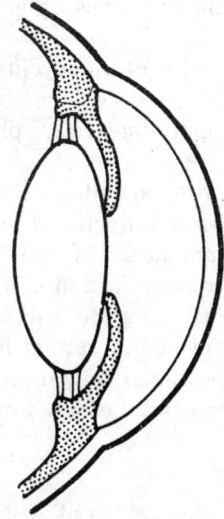

Fig. 7.4. Annular posterior synechia.

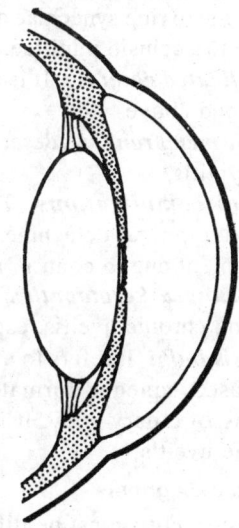

Fig. 7.5. Total posterior synechia causing deep anterior chamber.

6. Pupillary signs.
  i.   *Narrow irregular pupil.* Pupil is small, inactive and irregular due to synechia formation.
  ii. *Festooned pupil* refers to irregular dilation of pupil with mydriatics and is due to posterior synechia.
  iii. *Occlusio pupillae* refers to blocked or occlused pupil by the organized fibrous exudates.

7. Changes in the lens
  i.   *Pigment dispersal* on the anterior lens capsule is common.
  ii. *Exudates* may be deposited on the lens in acute plastic iridocyclitis.
  iii. *Complicated cataract* characterized by polychromatic lustre and bread-crumb appearance may occur in chronic cases.
  iv. *Cyclitic membrane* refers to organized exudates behind the lens.

8. Vitreous signs. Anterior vitreous may show exudates and inflammatory cells after an attack of uveitis.

Complications

1. Secondary glaucoma. It may occur as an early or late complication of iridocyclitis.
  – *Early glaucoma* (inflammatory glaucoma) occurs due to blockage of angle of anterior chamber with exudates.
  – *Late glaucoma* (postinflammatory glaucoma) is the result of pupil block

either due to ring synechiae and iris bombe formation (seclusio pupillae) or due to occlusio pupillae.

2. *Complicated cataract.* It is a common complication of iridocyclitis, as described above.

3. *Cyclitic membrane.* As described, it is a late complication of acute plastic iridocyclitis.

4. *Retinal complications.* These include cystoid macular oedema, exudative retinal detachment due to choroiditis and tractional retinal detachment due to contraction of cyclitic membrane .

5. *Band-shaped keratopathy.* It may occur as a complication of long-standing chronic uveitis, especially in children having Still's disease.

6. *Phthisis bulbi.* It refers to a soft and shrunken eyeball. It results due to decreased aqueous formation following from disorganization and atrophy of ciliary body. It is the final stage end result of any form of chronic uveitis.

Differential diagnosis

Acute iridocyctitis must be differentiated from other causes of acute red eye especially acute congestive glaucoma and acute conjunctivitis (Table 7.1).

Table 7.1: Distinguishing features of acute conjunctivitis, acute iridocyclitis and acute congestive glaucoma.

	Feature	*Acute Conjunctivitis*	*Acute Iridocyclitis*	*Acute congestive glaucoma*
1.	Onset	Gradual	Usually gradual	Sudden
2.	Pain	Mild discomfort	Moderate in eye and along the first division of trigeminal nerve	Severe in eye and the entire trigeminal area.
3.	Discharge	Mucopurulent	Watery	Watery
4.	Coloured halos	May be present	Absent	Present
5.	Vision	Good	Slightly impaired	Markedly impaired
6.	Congestion	Superficial conjunctival	Deep ciliary	Deep ciliary
7.	Tenderness	Absent	Marked	Marked
8.	Pupil	Normal	Small and irregular	Large and vertically oval.
9.	Media	Clear	Hazy due to KPs, aqueous flare and pupillary exudates.	Hazy due to edematous cornea.
10.	Anterior chamber	Normal	May be deep.	Very shallow
11.	Iris	Normal	Muddy	Oedematous
12.	Intraocular pressure	Normal	Usually normal	Raised
13.	Constitutional symptoms	Absent	Little	Prostration and vomiting.

Investigations

1. *Haematological investigations*
- Routine haemogram including TLC, DLC and ESR.
- Blood sugar to rule out diabetes mellitus.
- Serological tests for syphilis, toxoplasmosis, histoplasmosis, Rh factor, antinuclear antibodies and HLA typing.
2. *Urine examination* for RBC, WBC, pus cells and culture to rule out urinary tract infection.
3. *Stool examination* to rule out parasitic infestations.
4. *X-rays* of chest, paranasal sinuses, sacroiliac joint and lumbar spine.
5. *Skin-tests.* Mantoux test for tuberculosis and Kveim test for sarcoidosis.

Treatment

I. *Non-specific treatment*

A. *Local therapy*

1. *Atropine* (1%) eye drops or ointment instilled 3 times a day or other cycloplegic drugs are very useful and most effective drugs for iridocyclitis. Atropine helps in four ways:
- Gives comfort and rest to the eye by paralysing the ciliary muscle,
- Dilates the pupil and prevents or breaks the posterior synechia.
- Decreases hyperaemia and thus reduces exudation.
- Increases blood supply and thus more antibodies are brought in.

2. *Corticosteroids* are used or eyedrops 4-6 times in day and ointment at bed time or even as subconjunctival injection in severe cases. These are very effective due to their anti-inflammatory, antiallergic and antifibrotic effects. Commonly used topical steroid preparations are hydrocortisone acetate (0.5%), dexamethasone (0.1%) and betamethasone (1%).

3. *Non-steroidal anti-inflammatory* eye drops such as diclofenac, indomethacin, ketorolac or flurbiprofen may be used 4-6 times a day where corticosteroids are contraindicated.

B. *Systemic therapy*

1. *Systemic corticosteroids* are very useful in severe cases of iridocyclitis.
2. *Nonsteroidal anti-inflamatory* drugs (NSAIDs) such as diclofenac, aspirin or oxyphenbutazone relieve pain and inflammation.
3. *Sytemic ACTH* (adrenocorticotropic hormone) may be required in severe non-responsive cases.
4. *Immunosuppressive drugs* such as cyclophosphamide are used only in desparate and extremely serious cases of uveitis.

C. Physical measures

1. *Hot fomentation,* performed 3-4 times a day is very soothing. It diminishes pain and increases circulation.
2. *Dark goggles* give comfort by reducing photophobia.

II. Specific treatment

Specific treatment for the diseases such as tuberculosis, syphilis, toxoplasmosis etc must be given when detected.

POSTERIOR UVEITIS

Posterior uveitis refers to inflammation of the choroid (choroiditis). Because of close proximity, inflammation of choroid almost always involves the adjoining retina, and the resultant lesion is called chorioretinitis.

Etiology

Etiology of choroiditis is same as described for uveitis in general.

Clinical features

Depending upon site and number of lesions, choroiditis can be classified into :

1. *Diffuse choroiditis* i.e. involvement of almost whole of the choroid usually tubercular or syphilitic in nature.
2. *Disseminated choroiditis* is characterized by multiple but small areas of inflammation scattered over greater part of choroid.
3. *Central choroiditis.* It involves the central or macular area.
4. *Juxtapapillary choroiditis.* The lesions are present near the optic disc.

Symptoms. Choroiditis is a painless condition usually characterized by following visual symptoms :

1. *Defective vision* is mild due to vitreous haze, but may be severe in central choroiditis.
2. *Black spots floating in front of the eyes* occur due to exudates in the vitreous.
3. *Metamorphopsia, micropsia or macropsia* are the visual symptoms in which an object is seen as distorted, small in size or larger in size, respectively.

Signs. Usually there are no external signs and the eye looks quite. Fundus examination depending upon the type of choroiditis, may reveal localised, disseminated or diffuse patches of choroiditis. A patch of active choroiditis appears as a poli-yellow or dirty white raised area with ill defined margins. Lesion is typically deeper to retinal vessels. Overlying retina is oedematous and vitreous is hazy due to ulceration.

Treatment

It is broadly on the lines of anterior uveitis. Systemic corticorteroids constitute the main treatment.

SPECIFIC UVEITIS SYNDROMES

Fuch's uveitis syndrome

Fuch's heterochromic iridocyclitis is a chronic low grade anterior uveitis. It typically occurs in middle aged persons and involves only one eye. It is characterized by following features :

- Heterochromia of iris.
- Diffuse stromal iris atrophy
- Fine KPs at back of cornea
- Faint aqueous flare
- Absence of posterior synechia
- Complicated cataract is common

Glaucomatocyclitic crisis

It is also known as Posner-Schlossman syndrome. It typically affects young adults and is characterized by :

- Recurrent attacks of acute rise of intraocular pressure (40-50 mm of Hg)
- Fine KPs at the back of cornea
- Epithelial corneal oedema
- Dilated pupil and no posterior synechiae.
- A white eye (no congestion)

Sympathetic ophthalmitis

It is a rare bilateral granulomatous panuveitis which is known to occur following peneterating ocular trauma usually associated with incarceration of the uveal tissue in the wound. The injured eye is called 'exciting eye and the fellow eye which also develops uveitis is called' sympathising eye'. For details see page 192.

Pars planitis

Pars planitis (intermediate uveitis) denotes idiopathic inflammation of pars plana part of the ciliary body and most peripheral part of the retina. Patient may have history of floaters or defective vision. Externally eye looks quite. Fundus examination with indirect ophthalmoscope may show snow ball whitish exudates near the ora serrata in the inferior quadrant.

Behcet's syndrome

It is an idiopathic multisystem disease characterised by :
1. Recurrent iridocyclitis associated with hypopyon.
2. Ulcerative lesions on oral and genital mucosa.
3. Erythema multiforme.
4. Neurological and articular involvement may be associated.

Reiter's disease

It is an idiopathic condition which occurs in young males who are positive for HLA-B27. It is characterized by a triad of urethritis, arthritis and conjunctivitis. Iridocyclitis is associated in 20-30 percent cases.

Vogt-Koyanagi-Harada's (VKH) syndrome

It is an idiopathic multisystem disorder characterized by following features:

1. *Cutaneous lesions* : alopecia, poliosis and vitligo.
2. *Neurological lesions* : menigism, encephalitis tinnitis, vertigo, deafness.
3. *Ocular lesions* : chronic granulomatous anterior uveitis, posterior uveitis and exudative retinal detachment.

PURULENT ENDOPHTHALMITIS

Endophthalmitis is purulent infection of the inner structures of the eye ball which include the whole uveal tissue, retina, vitreous humour and aqueous humour.

Etiology

Common causative bacteria for purulent endophthalmitis are staphylococci, *Pseudomonas, E. coli,* pneumococci and streptococci. These organisms can enter the eyeball by following modes:

1. *Exogenous infection* following perforating injuries, ocular operations or perforation of corneal ulcer are the most common.
2. *Endogenous infection* through blood stream may occur due to metastasis of the infected embolus in the retinal artery and choroidal vessels.
3. *Secondary infection* from the surrounding infections such as orbital cellulitis is very rare.

Clinical picture

Symptoms include severe ocular pain, redness, lacrimation, photophobia and loss of vision.

Signs of bacterial endophthalmitis are :

1. *Lids* become red and swollen.
2. *Conjunctiva* shows chemosis and marked circumcorneal congestion.
3. *Cornea* is oedematous, cloudy and ring infiltration may be formed.
4. In exogenous form, edges of wound become yellow and necrotic.
5. *Anterior chamber* shows hypopyon, soon it becomes full of pus.
6. *Iris,* when visible is oedematous and muddy.
7. *Pupil* shows yellow reflex due to purulent exudation in vitreous. When anterior chamber becomes full of pus, iris and pupil details are not seen.
8. In metastatic forms and in cases with deep infections, posterior segment is first involved. Soon a yellowish white mass is seen through fixed dilated pupil. This sign is called *amaurotic cat's eye reflex.*
9. *Intraocular pressure* is raised in early stages, but in severe cases, the ciliary processes are destroyed, and a fall in intraocular pressure may ultimately result in shrinkage of the globe.

Treatment

Endophthalmitis is an emergency, therefore an early diagnosis and treatment is essential to save the eye.

I. Medical treatment

1. *Antibiotics.* To control the infection modern antibiotics such as amikacin, cefazoline, vancomycetin and tobramycin should be given immediately by following routes.
   - intravitreal injection,
   - subconjunctival injection,
   - fortified eye drops topically
   - systemic administration by intravenous and oral routes.
2. *Corticosteroids.* They have an anti-inflammatory action and to preserve ocular structures, their administration is essential. They should be used as topical drops, sub-conjunctival injection and oral tablets.
3. *Atropine* used as 1% drops and ointment is very useful (as described in treatment of iridocyclitis).

II. Surgical treatment

1. *Vitrectomy.* It should be performed to save the eye if the patient does not respond to medical therapy within 48 hours.
2. *Enucleation* i.e. removal of the eyeball is indicated only in patients with very painful and blind eye where all other measures have failed.

PANOPHTHALMITIS

It is an intense purulent inflammation of the whole eyeball including the Tenon's capsule. The disease usually begins either as purulent anterior or posterior uveitis; and soon a fullfledged picture of panophthalmitis develops, following through a very short stage of endophthalmitis.

Etiology

It is same as described for endophthalmitis.

Clinical picture

Symptoms : These include, severe ocular pain and headache, complete loss of vision, profuse watering, purulent discharge; marked redness and swelling of the eyes. Associated constitutional symptoms are malaise and fever.

Signs

1. *Lids* show a marked oedema and hyperaemia.
2. *Eyeball* is slightly proptosed, ocular movements are limited and painful.
3. *Conjunctiva* shows marked chemosis and ciliary as well as conjunctival congestion.
4. *Cornea* is cloudy and oedematous.
5. *Anterior chamber* is full of pus.
6. Vision is completely lost and perception of light is absent.

7. *Intraocular pressure* is markedly raised.
8. *Globe perforation* may occur at limbus, pus comes out and intraocular pressure falls.

Treatment

There is little hope of saving such an eye, and the pain and toxaemia lend an urgency to its removal.

1. To relieve pain, anti-inflammatory and analgesics should be started immediately.
2. To prevent further spread of infection in the surrounding structures broad spectrum antibiotics should be administered.
3. *Evisceration* operation should be performed to avoid the risk of intracranial dissemination of infection. Frill evisceration is preferred over conventional evisceration.

TUMOURS OF THE UVEAL TRACT

The commonest benign tumour of the uveal tract is the *naevus* and the most important tumour to be considered is *malignant melanoma*. Malignant melanoma arises from the neural crest derived pigment cells of the uvea as a solitary tumour and is usually unilateral. It may arise from a pre-existing naevus or denovo from the mature melanocytes present in the stroma. The commonest site of malignant melanoma is the choroid and next is the ciliary body and the iris.

MALIGNANT MELANOMA OF CHOROID

It is the most common primary intraocular tumour of adults, usually seen between 40-70 years of age.

Pathology

It consists of cells containing melanin pigment with reticulin fibres in the stroma. Depending upon cellular features, melanomes are six types.

1. *Spindle-A melanoma* is composed of small spindle-shaped cells.
2. *Spindle-B melanoma* comprises of large and plump spindle cells.
3. *Fascicular melanoma* is composed of either spindle-A or -B cells arranged in a pallisading manner.
4. *Epitheloid cell melanoma* consists of large oval or round pleomorphic cells.
5. *Mixed cell melanomas* are composed of both spindle and epitheloid cells.
6. *Necrotic melanomas* have massive tumour necrosis. The actual cell type cannot be recognised.

Clinical picture

It can be divided in four stages :

1. *Quiescent stage* is painless. Patient may have defective vision. Fundus

examination may show elevated tumour mass with an orange patch due to accumulation of lipofuscin. Large tumour produces exudative retinal detachment.

2. *Glaucomatous stage* is characterized by severe pain, redness, total loss of vision and stony hard eye.
3. *Stage of extraocular extension* occurs after the progressive tumour growth bursts through the sclera usually near the limbus. It is followed by rapid fungation and orbital invasion with proptosis (Fig.7.6).
4. *Stage of distant metastasis* usually the metastasis is blood-borne to the liver and central nervous system.

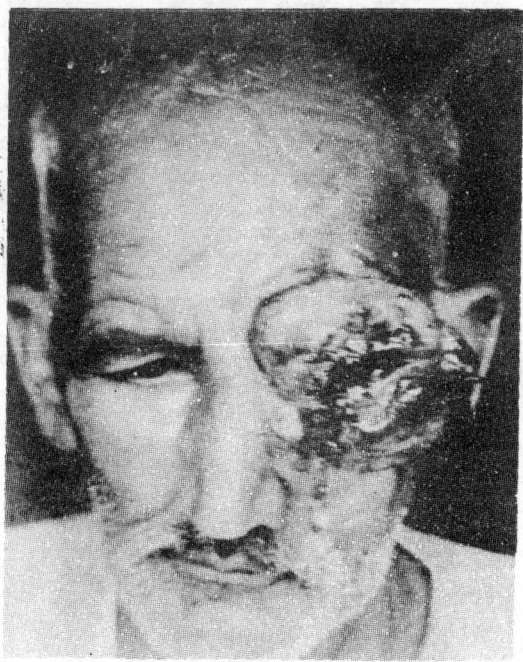

Fig. 7.6. Fungating malignant melanoma of the choroid involving orbit.

Treatment

Small tumours (under 7 mm) may be treated conservatively using cobalt plaques or photocoagulation. However, usually it is best to enucleate the eyeball as early as possible.

8

Diseases of the Lens

CATARACT

The normal crystalline lens is a transparent structure. Occurrence of any opacity in the lens or its capsule whether developmental or acquired is called cataract.

Classification

A. Etiological classification

 I. Congenital and developmental cataract

 II. Acquired cataract

   1. Senile cataract

   2. Traumatic cataract

   3. Complicated cataract

   4. Metabolic cataract

   5. Electric cataract

   6. Radiational cataract

   7. Toxic cataract e.g.

     i. Corticosteroid-induced cataract

     ii. Miotics-induced cataract

     iii. Copper (in chalcosis) and iron (in siderosis) induced cataract.

   8. Cataract associated with skin diseases (dermatogenic cataract).

   9. Cataract associated with osseous diseases.

  10. Cataract with miscellaneous syndromes e.g.

     i. Dystrophica myotonica

     ii. Down's syndrome.

B. Morphological classification (Fig. 8.1)

1. *Capsular cataract.* It involves the capsule and may be:

   i. Anterior capsular cataract

   ii. Posterior capsular cataract

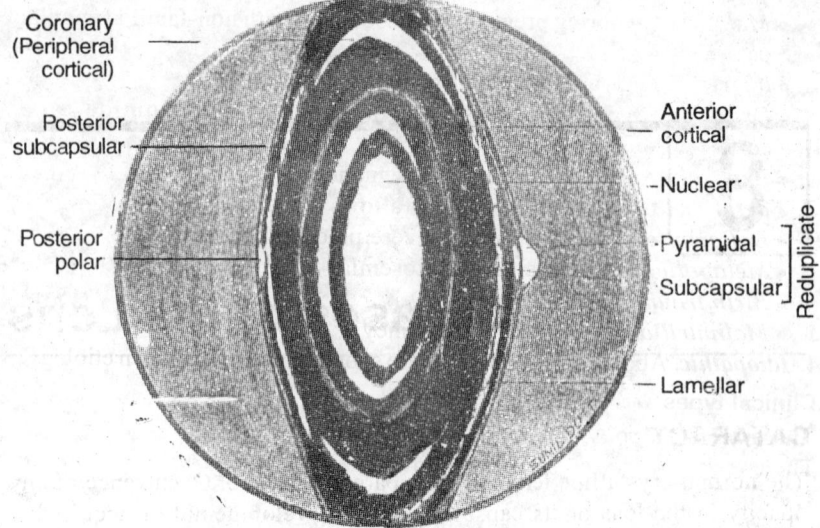

Fig. 8.1. Morphological shapes of cataract.

2. *Subcapsular cataract.* It involves the superficial part of the cortex (just below the capsule) and includes:
   i. Anterior subcapsular cataract
   ii. Posterior subcapsular cataract
3. *Cortical cataract.* It involves the major part of the cortex.
4. *Supranuclear cataract.* It involves only the deeper parts of cortex (just outside the nucleus).
5. *Nuclear cataract.* It involves the nucleus of the crystalline lens.
6. *Polar cataract.* It involves the capsule and superficial part of the cortex in the polar region only and may be:
   i. Anterior polar cataract
   ii. Posterior polar cataract

CONGENITAL AND DEVELOPMENTAL CATARACT

These occur due to some disturbance in the normal growth of the lens. When disturbance occurs before birth, the child is born with a *congenial cataract.* The *developmemntal cataract* occurs from infancy to adolescence. It is impotant to note that congenital and developmental cataract typically affect a particular zone which is being formed when the disturbance occurs.

Etiology

1. *Heredity.* About one-third of all congenital cataracts are hereditary.

2. *Maternal factors* which play a role are :

- *Malnutrition* during pregnancy is associated with non-familial zonular cataract.
- *Infections* e.g. rubella in the first trimester.
- *Drug ingestion* during pregnancy e.g. thalidomide and corticosteroids.
- *Exposure to radiations* during pregnancy.

3. *Foetal or infantile factors* are as follows :
- *Deficient oxygenation* due to severe placental haemorrhage.
- *Metabolic disorders* e.g., galactosemia.
- *Birth trauma*
- *Malnutrition* during early pregnancy

4. *Idiopathic.* About 50 percent cases are sporadic and of unknown etiology.

Clinical types

There are numerous varities of congenital and developmental cataracts. The common one are described below :

1. *Punctate or blue dot cataract.* It is characterized by tiny bluish-white multiple punctate opacities scattered all over the lens. These opacities are stationary and do not affect vision.

2. *Zonular or lamellar cataract.* It is the most common variety. It is usually bilateral with a strong hereditary tendency. It may also occur due to malnutrition and deficiency of vitamin D in the mother.

Zonular cataract, typically occurs in the zone of foetal nucleus surrounding the embryonic nucleus (Fig.8.2), and is associated with severe visual loss.

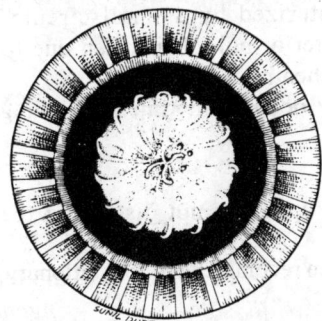 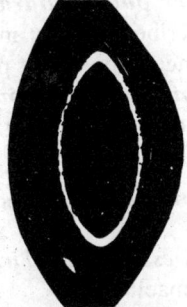

(A) by oblique illumination;   (B) in optical section with the
                                         beam of the slit-lamp.

Fig. 8.2. Lamellar (zonular) cataract as seen

3. *Sutural cataract.* It is characterized by presence of a series of punctate opacities scattered around the anterior and posterior Y-sutures. Such cataracts are usually stationary, bilateral and cause no visual disturbance.

4. *Coronary cataract.* It is a common form of developmental cataract occuring during puberty and thus involving either the adolescent nucleus or deeper layers of the cortex (Fig. 8.3). It is characterized by multiple club-shaped opacities near the periphery of the lens which are hidden by the iris and usually do not cause visual disturbance.

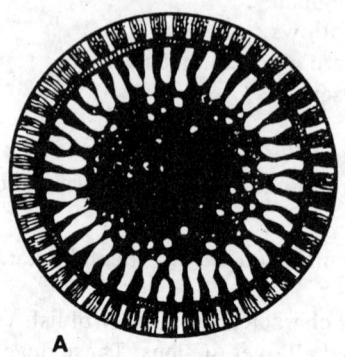
A

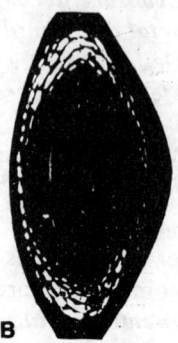
B

Fig. 8.3. Coronary cataract as seen (A) by oblique illumination; (B) in optical section with the beam of the slit-lamp.

5. *Total congenital cataract.* It is a common variety and may be unilateral or bilateral. Usually the child is born with a dense white opacity.
6. *Anterior polar cataract.* It may occur due to delayed formation of anterior chamber or corneal perforation in early pregnancy.
7. *Posterior polar cataract.* It is characterized by a small circular circumscribed opacity involving the posterior pole. It is often due to persistence of posterior part of vascular sheath.
8. *Congenital membranous cataract* may occur sometimes following absorption of congenital cataract.

Treatment

1. *No treatment* is required for stationary opacities not disturbing the vision.
2. *Mydriactics and optical iridectomy* has been recommended for stationary central opacities.
3. *Extracapsular cataract extraction* with intraocular lens implantation is the surgical treatment of choice for all childhood cataracts impairing vision.

ACQUIRED CATARACT

SENILE OR AGE-RELATED CATARACT

It is the commonest form of acquired cataract. It affects equally persons of either sex usually above the age of 50 years. Classically the senile cataract occurs in two forms, the cortical (soft cataract) and nuclear (hard cataract). The cortical cataract may start as cuneiform (more common) or cupuliform cataract. It is common to find nuclear and cortical senile cataract existing in the same eye.

Etiology

Senile cataract is essentially an ageing process. Various factors implicated in its etiopathogensis are as follows :

A. Factors affecting age of onset, type and maturation of senile cataract
1. Heredity
2. Exposure to ultraviolet irradiation
3. Dietary deficiency of certain essential elements
4. Dehydrational crisis in childhood.

B. Mechanism of loss of transparency. It is basically different in cortical and nuclear senile cataract.
1. *Cortical senile cataract* is associated with following biochemical changes :
   - *Hydration* occurs due to electrolytic imbalance: Lens fibres swell up and become opaque.
   - *Denaturation and coagulation* of lens proteins leads to formation of dense irrevesible lenticular opacity.
2. *Nuclear senile cataract* occurs due to intensification of sclerotic changes associated with dehydration and compaction of the nucleus. There occurs pigmentation due to deposition of urochrome and melanin derived from the amino acids in the lens.

Stages of maturation

A. Maturation of senile cortical cataract shows following stages :
1. *Stage of lamellar separation* refers to demarcation of cortical fibres due to their separation by fluid vacuoles. These changes are reversible.
2. *Stage of incipient cataract* is characterized by formation of early detectable opacities with clear areas in between. In *cuneiform type of cataract* wedge opacities start from the equator; while in cupuliform cataract opacities start in the central part as posterior subcapsular cataract.
3. *Immature senile cataract (ISC).* In this stage opacification progresses involving deeper layers of cortex. In some cases lens fibres may swell markedly leading to formation of *intumescent cataract.*
4. *Mature senile cataract (MSC).* In this stage entire cortex is opacified. (Pl III.2)
5. *Hypermature senile cataract (HMSC).* Hypermaturity may occur in any of the two forms:

(a) *Morgagnian hypermature cataract* develops when the entire cortex is liquified and the lens is converted into a bag of milky fluid. The small brown nucleus settles at the bottom.

(b) *Sclerotic type of hypermature cataract* is characterized by a shrunken lens (due to leakage of water) with wrinkled and thickened anterior capsule.

B. Maturation of senile nuclear cataract. During maturation of nuclear cataract the nucleus may become diffusely cloudy (greyish) or tinted yellow to black) due to deposition of pigment. In clinical practice the commonly observed pigmented nuclear cataracts are either amber, brown (cataract brunescens) or black (cataract nigra) and very rarely red (cataracta rubra) in colour.

Clinical features

Symptoms. Common symptoms of senile cataract are glare, uniocular polyopia, coloured halos, black spots infront of the eyes, and gradual progressive loss of vision.

Signs of senile cataract are summarised in Table 8.1.

Complications

Complications of untreated senile cataract include phacomorphic glaucoma, phacoanaphylactic glaucoma, phacoanaphylactic uveitis and subluxation or dislocation of the lens.

OTHER ACQUIRED CATARACTS

Metabolic cataracts

1. **Diabetic cataract.** The true diabetic cataract is characterized by 'snow-flake' opacities, usually occurring in young adults. Accumulation of 'sorbital' is primarily responsible for development of a true diabetic cataract.

2. **Galactosaemic cataract.** Galactosaemic cataract is associated with inborn error of galactose metabolism due to deficiency of galactose-1- phosphate uridyltransferase (GPUT). A related disorder occurs due to deficiency of galactokinase. Accumulation of 'dulcitol' is primarily responsible for development of galactosaemic cataract. Development of cataract may be prevented by early diagnosis and elimination of milk from the diet.

3. **Hypocalcaemic cataract.** Hypocalcaemic cataract may be associated with parathyroid tetany.

4. **Sunflower cataract.** Sunflower cataract may be associated with inborn error of copper metabolism (Wilson's disease).

5. **Cataract in Lowe's syndrome.** Cataract may be seen in Lowe's (oculo-cerebral-renal) syndrome; an inborn error of amino-acid metabolism.

Table 8.1: Signs of senile cataract

Examination	Nuclear cataract	ISC	MSC	HMSC(M)	HMSC(S)
1. Visual acuity	6/9 to PL+	6/9 to FC+	HM+ to PL+	PL+	PL+
2. Colour of lens	Grey, amber, brown, black or red	Greyish white	Pearly white	Milky white with sinking brownish nucleus	Dirty white with hyper-white spots leus
3. Iris shadow	Seen	Seen	Not seen	Not seen	Not seen
4. Distant direct ophthalmoscopy with dilated pupil	Central dark area against red fundal glow	Multiple dark areas against red fundal glow	No red glow but white pupil due to complete cataract	No red glow milky white pupil	No red glow
5. Slit-lamp examination	Nuclear opacity clear cortex	Areas of normal with cataractous cortex	Complete cortex is cataractous	Milky white sunken brownish nucleus	Shrunken cataract lens with thickened anterior capsule

ISC: Immature senile cataract, MSC: Mature senile cataract, HMSC (M) Hypermature senile cataract (Morgagnian), HMSC (S): Hypermature senile cataract (Sclerotic), PL: Perception of light, HM: Hand movements, FC: Finger counting.

Complicated cataract

Etiology. It may occur secondary to uveitis, retinitis pigmentosa, myopic chorio-retinal degeneration and long standing retinal detachment.

Clinical features

Posterior subcapsular cataract is typically characterised by polychromatic lustre and bread crumb appearance.

Toxic cataracts

1. *Corticosteroid induced cataract.* Posterior subcapsular opacities may be associated with the use of topical as well as systemic steroids.

2. *Miotics induced cataract.* Anterior subcapsular granular cataract may be associated with the use of long acting miotics such as echothiophate and demecarium bromide.

Radiational cataract

1. *Infra-red (heat) cataract.* It typically occurs as discoid posterior subcapsular opacities in workers of glass industry, hence the name 'glass-blower's cataract'.

2. *Irradiation cataract.* It may follow exposure to X-rays, gamma-rays of neutron.

3. *Ultraviolet radiation.* Ultraviolet radiation has been linked with senile cataract.

Electric cataract

It may occur following passage of powerful electric current through the body.

Syndermatotic cataract

It is associated with skin disorders like atopic dermatitis, scleroderma and keratosis.

MANAGEMENT OF CATARACT IN ADULTS

Indications of surgery

1. *Visual impairment*
2. Medical indications include phacomorphic glaucoma, phacolytic glaucoma and associated diabetic retinopathy or retinal detachment which needs treatment.
3. *Cosmetic indication i.e.* removal of white cataract in order to obtain black pupil without any hope of getting useful vision.

Preoperative evaluation

1. *Ocular examination* should be performed to note:
a) Pupillary reactions
b) Visual acuity
c) Projection of light

d) Macular function tests
   – Two point discrimination test
   – Maddox rod test
   – Colour perception
e) Patency of lacrimal apparatus should be tested by syringing.
f) Intraocular pressure measurement.
2. *Systemic examination* to exclude diabetes mellitus, hypertension, cardiac problems, obstructive lung disorders and any potential source of infection in the body such as septic gums and urinary tract infection.

Choice of surgical technique

It depends upon following factors (In general ECCE is preferred over ICCE) :

1. *Age of the patient.* Below 40 years ICCE is contraindicated due to strong zonules.
2. *Surgical facilities and skill.* If facilities or skill for microsurgery is not available ICCE is performed.
3. *Quantum of surgical load.* In eye camps, where about 50 operations are performed per day by each surgeon, ICCE is preferred over ECCE.
4. *When posterior chamber* intraocular lens (IOL) is planned, ECCE is the choice.
5. *In high myopia.* ECCE should be preferred.
6. *In ubluxated lens.* ICCE is preferred.

Preoperative medications and preparations

1. *Topical antibiotics* such as tobramycin or gentamicin QID for 3 days just before surgery is advisable as prophylaxis against endophthalmitis.
2. *Systemic antibiotics* such as gentamicin 80 mg intramuscular at night and in the morning before surgery are preferred by a few surgeons..
3. *Preparation of the eye to be operated.* Eyelashes of upper lid should be trimmed at night and the eye to be operated should be marked.
4. *An informed and detailed consent* should be obtained.
5. *Scrub bath and care of hair.* Each patient should be instructed to have a scrub bath including face and hair wash with soap and water. Male patients must get their beard cleaned and hair trimmed. Female patients should comb their hair properly.
6. *To lower IOP,* acetazolamide 500 mg stat 2 hours before surgery and glycerol 60 ml mixed with equal amount of water or lemon juice, 1 hour before surgery, or intravenous mannitol 1 gm/kg body weight half an hour before surgery may be used.
7. *To sustain dilated pupil* (especially in extracapsular cataract extraction) the *antiprostaglandin eyedrops* such as indomethacin or flurbiprofen should be instilled three times one day before surgery and half hourly for two

hours immediately before surgery. Adequate dilation of pupil can be achieved by instillation of 1 percent *tropicamide* and 5 percent or 10 percent *phenylephrine* eyedrops every ten minutes, one hour before surgery.

Types of surgical technique

I. Intracapsular cataract extraction (ICCE)

In this technique (Fig. 8.4) entire lens with intact capsule is removed. Weak and degenerated zonules is a prerequisite for this method. Therefore, this technique cannot be employed in younger patients where zonules are strong. In ICCE lens can be delivered by different techniques namely, Indian Smith method, cryoextraction (Fig. 8.4F), and capsule forceps method.

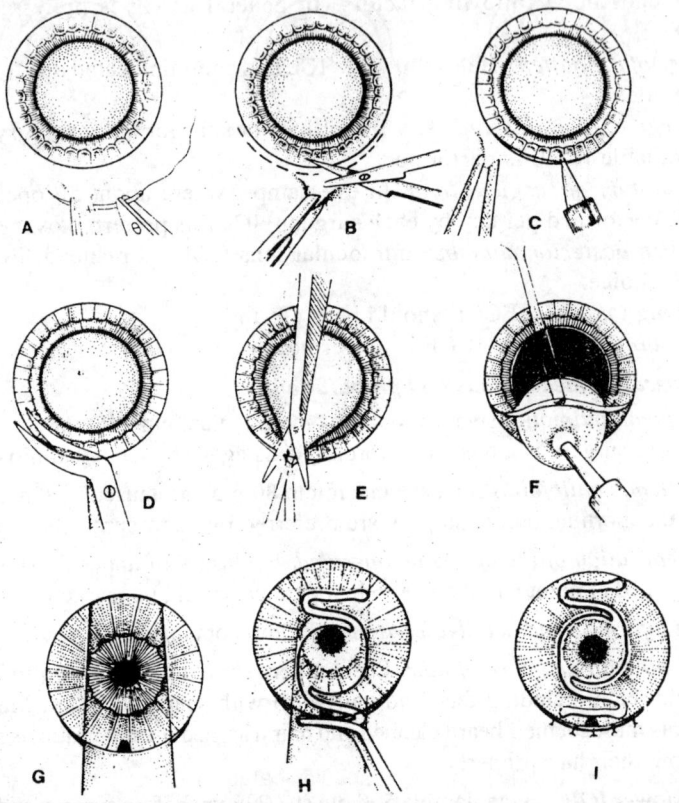

Fig. 8.4. Surgical steps of intracapsular cataract extraction with intraocular lens implantation: (A) passing of superior rectus suture; (B) fornix-based conjunctival flap; (C) partial thickness groove; (D) completion of corneo-scleral section; (E) peripheral iridectomy, (F) cryolens extraction; (G&H) insertion of Kelman multiflex intraocular lens in anterior chamber; (I) corneo-scleral suturing.

II. Extracapsular cataract extraction (ECCE)

In this technique, major portion of anterior capsule with epithelium, nucleus and cortex are removed leaving behind intact posterior capsule. Presently following methods of extracapsular cataract extraction are known:

1. *Conventional extracapsular cataract extraction (ECCE)* : Presently it is the operation of choice in almost all cataracts. It is performed under microscope. Its main steps are meticulous anterior capsulotomy, expression of nucleus and aspiration of cortex (Fig. 8.5).

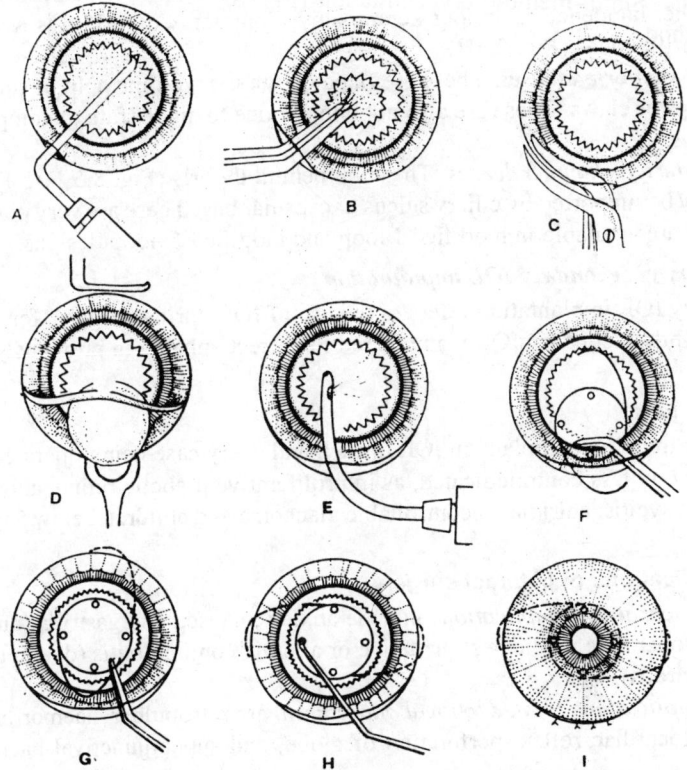

Fig. 8.5. Surgical steps of extracapsular cataract extraction with posterior chamber intraocular lens implantation: (A) anterior capsulotomy—can-opener's technique; (B) removal of anterior capsule; (C) completion of corneo-scleral section; (D) removal of nucleus (pressure and counter-pressure method); (E) aspiration of cortex; (F) insertion of inferior haptic of posterior chamber IOL; (G) insertion of superior haptic of PC-IOL; (H) dialing of the IOL; (I) corneo-scleral suturing.

2. *Phacoemulsification :* It is an advanced technique of ECCE. In it, after central anterior capsulotomy, nucleus is emulsified and aspirated by phacoemulsifier and the remaining cortical lens matter is aspirated with the help of an irrigating-aspiration cannula. The phaco needle vibrates longitudinally at an ultrasonic speed of 40,000 times per second.

Intraocular lens implantation

It is the best method for correction of aphakia.

Types

1. *Anterior chamber IOLs.* These lie entirely in front of the iris and are supported in the angle. These are not much popular due to comparatively higher incidence of bullous keratopathy. Commonly used IOL is Kelman multiflex lens (Fig. 8.4H).
2. *Iris supported lenses.* These are fixed on the iris with the help of sutures, loops or claws. These are also not popular due to higher rate of complications.
3. *Posterior chamber lenses.* These lie behind the iris (Fig. 8.5 F to I) and may be supported by ciliary sulcus or capsular bag. These are very popular and are available in modified J-loop and modified C-loop designs.

Primary vs secondary IOL implantation

Primary IOL implantation refers to the use of IOL during surgery for cataract; while secondary IOL is implanted to correct aphakia in previously operated eye.

Indications

Recent trend is to implant an IOL in each and every case being operated for cataract, unless contraindicated, as in proliferative diabetic retinopathy, recurrent uveitis, aniridia, uncontrollable glaucoma and children below 5 years of age.

Complications of cataract surgery

A. *Preoperative complications* include anxiety, nausea and gastritis (due to pre-operative medicines), irritative or allergic conjunctivitis (due to topical drops).
B. *Complications related to local anaesthesia* are retrobulbar haemorrhage, oculocardiac reflex, perforation of globe, and subconjunctival haemorrhage.
C. *Operative complications* include superior rectus muscle laceration, excessive bleeding during conjunctival flap, irregular corneoscleral section; inadvertent injury to the back of cornea or iris or lens, vitreous loss and expulsive choroidal haemorrhage.
D. *Early postoperative complications are :* hyphaema, iris prolapse, striate keratopathy, shallow anterior chamber, endophthalmitis.

E. *Late post-operative complications* include cystoid macular oedema (CME), aphakic retinal detachment, epithelial ingrowth, vitreous touch syndrome, fibrous downgrowth, and after cataract (membranous, Elschnig's pearls or Sommerring's ring).

F. *IOL related complications* are comparatively higher incidence of CME, uveitis, and secondary glaucoma. Malpositions of IOL include inferior subluxation (sunset syndrome), superior subluxation (sunrise syndrome) and lost lens syndrome. Toxic lens syndrome refers to lens related uveal inflammation.

Postoperative management and Nursing care

The aim during postoperative nursing care is to allow full healing of the wound. General principles of nursing care are described on page 41-44.

The postoperative management after cataract extraction is as follows :

1. The patient is asked to lie quietly upon the back for about three hours and advised to take nil orally.
2. For mild to moderate postoperative pain injection diclofenac sodium may be given.
3. Next morning bandage is removed and eye is inspected for any postoperative complication. Then eye is dressed with 1 drop of 1% cyclopentolate and antibiotic-steroid ointment. Daily dressing continues for about 3-4 days after which tinted glasses are advised.
4. Antibiotic-steroid eyedrops are continued for four times, three times, two times and then once a day for 2 weeks each.
5. After 4-6 weeks of operation corneoscleral sutures are removed.
6. Final spectacles are prescribed after about 8 weeks of operation.

DISPLACEMENTS OF THE LENS

Displacement of the lens from its normal position (in patellar fossa) results from partial or complete rupture of the lens zonules.

ETIOLOGY

I. *Congenital displacements*. These may occur in the following forms:
   (a) *Simple ectopia lentis*. In this condition displacement is bilaterally symmetrical and usually upwards.
   (b) *Ectopia lentis et pupillae*. It is characterised by displacement of the lens associated with slit-shaped pupil which is displaced in the opposite direction.
   (c) *Ectopia lentis with systemic anomalies*. Salient features of some common conditions are as follows:
      1. *Marfan's syndrome*. It is an autosomal dominant mesodermal dysplasia. In this condition lens is displaced upwards and temporally (bilaterally symmetrical). Systemic anomalies include arachnodactly (spider fin-

gers), long extremities, hyperextensibility of joints, high arched palate and dissecting aortic aneurysm.

2. *Homocystinuria.* It is an autosomal recessive, inborn error of metabolism. In it the lens is usually subluxated downwards and nasally.

3. *Weil-Marchesani syndrome.* It is condition of autosomal recessive mesodermal dysplasia. *Ocular features* are spherophakia, and forward subluxation of lens which may cause pupil block glaucoma. *Systemic features* are short stature, stubby fingers and mental retardation.

4. *Ehlers-Danlos syndrome.* In it the *ocular features* are subluxation of lens and blue sclera. The *systemic features* include hyperextensibility of joints and loose skin with folds.

II. Traumatic displacement of the lens. It is usually associated with concussion injuries.

TOPOGRAPHICAL TYPES

Topographically, displacements of the lens may be classified as subluxation and luxation or dislocation.

I. Subluxation

It is partial displacement in which lens is moved sideways (up, down, medially or laterally), but remains behind the pupil. It results from partial rupture or unequal stretching of the zonules.

II. Dislocation or luxation of the lens

In it all the zonules are severed from the lens. A dislocated lens may be incarcerated into the pupil or present in the anterior chamber, the vitreous (where it may be floating – *lens nutans;* or fixed to retina – *lens fixata),* subretinal space, subscleral space or extruded out of the globe, partially or completely.

9

Glaucoma

AQUEOUS HUMOUR AND INTRAOCULAR PRESSURE

The intraocular pressure (IOP) is influenced by the pressure of the vitreous in the posterior segment of the eye and aqueous filling the anterior chamber. Normally the vitreous volume remains constant and thus it is the aqueous which is mainly responsible for variations in the intraocular pressure. In other words the pathophysiology of glaucoma revolves around the aqueous humour dynamics. The principal ocular structures concerned with the formation and drainage of aqueous humour are ciliary body, angle of anterior chamber and aqueous out flow system (see page 4 & 7).

Aqueous humour

It is a clear watery fluid filling the anterior chamber (0.25 ml) and posterior chamber (0.6 ml) of the eyeball. It is derived from plasma within the capillary network of ciliary processes. The normal aqueous production rate is 2.3 µl/ min. The three mechanisms - diffusion, ultrafiltration and secretion (active transport) play a part in its production at different levels.

After being produced by the ciliary processes, the aqueous humour flows from the posterior chamber into the anterior chamber through the pupil (Fig. 9.1). From the anterior chamber the aqueous is drained out by two routes. Trabecular (conventional) outflow accounts for the 90 percent and uveoscleral out flow for the 10 percent.

The intraocular pressure

The intraocular pressure (IOP) refers to the pressure exerted by the intraocular contents on the coats of the eyeball. Normal IOP varies between 10 and 21 mm of Hg (mean 16 ± 5 mm of Hg). The normal level of IOP is essentially maintained by a dynamic equilibrium between the formation and outflow of the aqueous humour. Thus, an increase in IOP may occur due to an increase in the formation of the aqueous or a difficulty in its outflow. Of these, the first is of little importance in clinical practice. Hence, an increase in IOP is essentially due to an obstruction to the outflow of aqueous humour at any level starting from pupil to episcleral vessels.

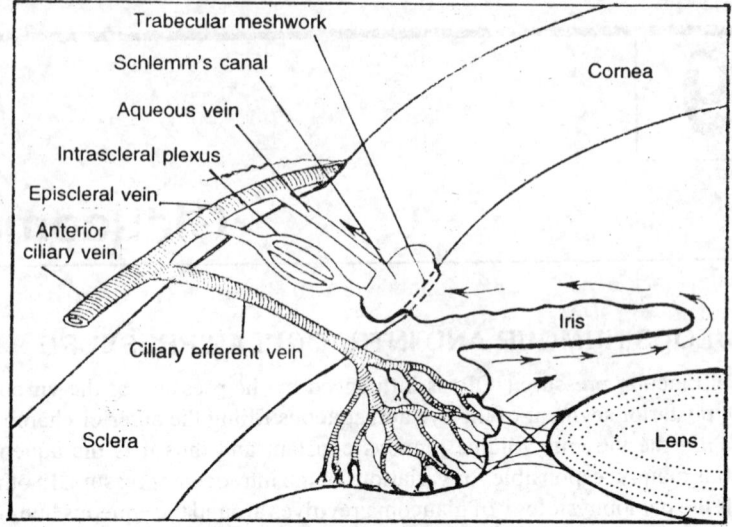

Fig. 9.1. The aqueous outflow system.

NOMENCLATURE AND CLASSIFICATION

Glaucoma is not a single disease process but a group of disorders in which intraocular pressure is raised above the tolerance limit of the affected eye, resulting in a damage to the optic nerve head and irreversible visual field defects.

This definition is not so simple as it apparently looks; since it is impossible to know the tolerance limit of the individual eye. Consequently the term *'ocular hypertension'* is used for cases having constantly raised IOP without any associated glaucomatous damage. Conversely, the term *normal* or *low tension glaucoma (NTG/LTG)* is suggested for the typical cupping of the disc and/or visual field defects associated with a normal or low IOP.

Classification

Clinico-etiologically glaucoma may be classified as follows:

(A) Congenital and developmental glaucomas
1. Primary congenital glaucoma (without associated anomalies).
2. Developmental glaucoma (with associated anomalies).

(B) Primary glaucomas
1. Primary open angle glaucoma (POAG)
2. Primary angle closure glaucoma (PACG)
3. Primary mixed mechanism glaucoma

(C) Secondary glaucomas

CONGENITAL / DEVELOPMENTAL GLACUOMA

It is characterized by elevation of intraocular pressure (IOP) associated with developmental abnormalities of the angle of anterior chamber.

Depending upon the age of onset the developmental glaucomas are termed as follows:

1. *True congenital glaucoma* is labelled when IOP is raised during intrauterine life and child is born with ocular enlargement. It occurs in about 40 percent of cases.

2. *Infantile glaucoma* is labelled when the disease manifests prior to the child's third birthday. It occurs in about 50 percent of cases.

3. *Juvenile glaucoma* is labelled in the rest 10 percent of cases who develop pressure rise between 3-16 years of life.

When the disease manifests prior to age of 3 years, the eyeball enlarges and so the term *'buphthalmos'* (bull-like eyes) is used. As it results due to retention of aqueous humour (watery solution), the term *'hydrophthalmos,* has also been suggested.

Clinical features

- Lacrimation (first symptom), photophobia, blepharospasm and eye rubbing.
- Buphthalmos (with onset before the age of 3 years), characterized by enlarged eyeball, corneal diameter more than 13 mm, corneal oedema (first sign), Haab's striae (healed splits in Descemet's membrane), deep anterior chamber, raised IOP, and variable optic disc cupping. Eye becomes myopic.
- *Gonioscopic examination* may reveal : Mesodermal membrane (Barkan's membrane), thinkening of trabecular sheets, hypoplastic iris stroma and insertion of iris above scleral spur.

Evaluation

A complete examination under general anaesthesia should be performed on each child suspected of having congenital glaucoma. The examination should include following:

1. *Measurement of IOP* with Schiotz or preferably hand-held Perkin's applanation tonometer since scleral rigidity is very low in children.
2. *Measurement of corneal diameter* by callipers.
3. *Ophthalmoscopy* to evaluate optic disc.
4. *Gonioscopic examination* of angle of anterior chamber reveals trabeculodysgenesis with either flat or concave iris insertion as described in pathogenesis.

Treatment

It is primarily surgical. However, IOP must be lowered by use of hyperosmotic agents, acetazolamide and beta-blocker eye drops till following surgery is taken up :

1. *Goniotomy.* In this operation an incision is made in the angle of anterior chamber under gonioscopic control (Fig. 9.2).

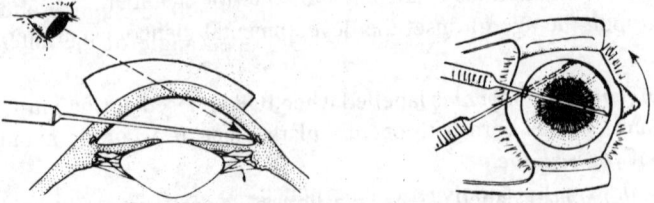

A. Position of goniotomy knife in the angle under direct visualization.

B. Procedure of sweeping of knife in the angle.

Fig. 9.2. Technique of goniotomy.

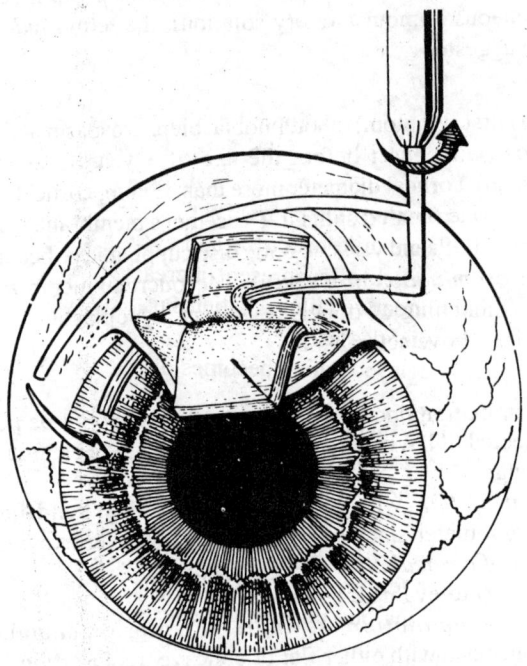

Fig. 9.3. Technique of trabeculotomy.

2. *Trabeculotomy.* In this procedure the angle of anterior chamber is opened with the help of an instrument the Hem's trabeculotome passed in the Schlemm's canal from outside (Fig. 9.3).
3. *Combined trabeculectomy and trabeculotomy* is now-a-days the preferred surgery with better results.

PRIMARY GLAUCOMAS

PRIMARY OPEN ANGLE GLAUCOMA

It is characterized by raised IOP associated with optic disc cupping and/or field defects, in an otherwise normal eye with open angle of the anterior chamber.

Etiology

Predisposing and risk factors

1. *Heredity.* POAG has a polygenic inheritance.
2. *Age.* It affects about 1 in 200 of population over 40 years of age. Risk increases in 50-70 years of age.
3. High myopes, diabetics and patients with thyrotoxicosis are more predisposed than the normal population.

Pathogenesis

IOP is raised due to decreased aqueous outflow facility resulting from thickening and sclerosis of the trabeculae and changes in the endothelial lining of the canal of Schlemm.

Clinical features

Symptoms

1. The disease is slowly progressive and usually asymptomatic, until it has caused a significant loss of visual field.
2. Patient may experience mild headache and eyeache.
3. Reading and close work often present increasing difficulties owing to progressive accommodative failure. Patients usually complain of frequent changes in presbyopic glasses.
4. Dark adaptation is delayed which becomes disturbing in later stages.

Signs

1. *IOP changes.* Initially there is exaggeration of the normal diurnal variation. A difference of more than 6 mm observed on repeated (every 4 hours) testing of IOP for 24 hours is suspicious and over 8 is diagnostic (normal, below 5 mm Hg).
2. *Cupping of the optic disc.* A slowly progressive cupping of the optic disc is an essential feature of POAG. Normal cup disc ratio is 0.3 (Fig. 9.4A). Glaucomatous cupping of the disc (Fig. 9.4B ot D) has following features:
   i. *Vertically oval cup* occurs due to selective loss of neural tissue in inferior and superior poles.
   ii. *Asymmetry of the cups,* a difference of more than 0.2 between two eyes is significant.
   iii. *Nasal shift* of blood vessels at the disc.
   iv. *Marked cupping* (0.7 to 0.9) may occur in advanced cases.

v. *Glaucomatous optic atrophy* (white and deep excavated disc is the end result).

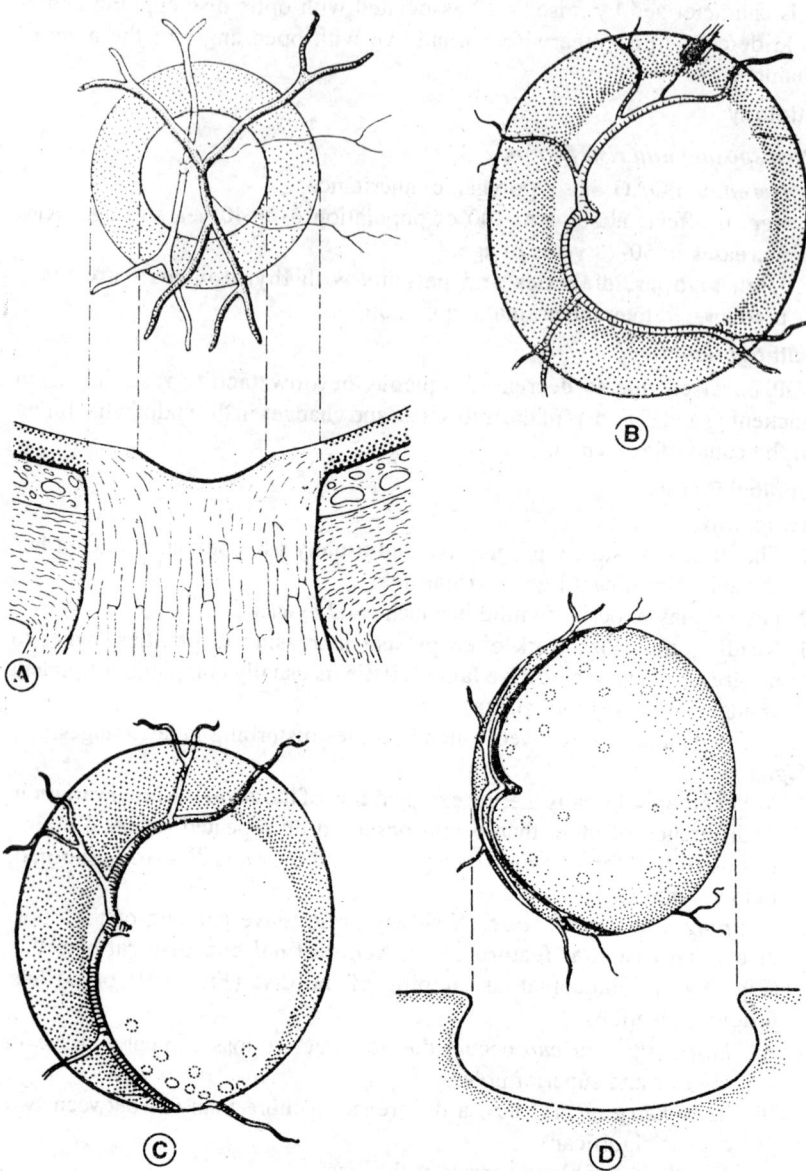

Fig. 9.4. Optic disc: (A) normal; (B) early glaucomatous changes; (C) advanced glaucomatous changes; (D) glaucomatous optic atrophy.

3. *Visual field defects* (Fig.9.5) These run parallel to the optic disc changes and progress in the following sequence :
   - Baring of blind spot (earliest field defect).
   - Paracentral scotoma between 10-20 degrees of visual field (Bjerrum's area).
   - Seidel's sign (sickle-shaped extension of blind spot).
   - Arcuate or Bjerrum's scotoma.
   - Ring or double arcuate scotoma.
   - Roenne's central nasal step.
   - Peripheral nasal step of Roenne's.
   - Tubular vision with a temporal island of vision.
   - Advanced field loss with a temporal island of vision only.
   - Complete loss of vision.

Diagnosis

Depending upon the levels of IOP, disc changes and visual field defects, the patients are assigned to one of the following diagnostic entities :

1. *Established POAG :* IOP more than 23 mmHg associated with definite disc cupping and visual field defects.
2. *POAG :* IOP more than 23 mm Hg with either disc changes or field defects.
3. *Glaucoma suspect or ocular hypertension:* IOP more than 23 mmHg with no disc changes or visual field defects.
4. *Low tension glaucoma (LTG)* or Normal tension glaucoma : IOP less than 21 mmHg with typical disc and/or visual field defects.

Treatment

1. *Medical therapy.* The initial therapy of POAG is still medical with surgery as the last resort. Commonly used antiglaucoma drugs are as follows:
   i. *Topical beta-blockers.* There are being recommended as the first drug of choice for medical therapy of POAG. These lower the IOP by reducing the aqueous secretion due to their effect as beta receptors in the ciliary processes. Preparations of beta-blockers in use are :
      - Timolol maleate (0.25, 0.5%; 1-2 times/day)
      - Betaxolol (0.25%, 2 times/day)
      - Levobunolol (0.25, 0.5%, 1-2 times/day).
   ii. *Pilocarpine* (1, 2, 4%, 3-4 times/day). It had remained the sheet anchor in the medical management POAG till recently. It lowers the IOP by increasing aqueous outflow by opening spaces in the trabecular meshwork in patients with POAG. Presently it is considered as an adjunctive therapy where other combinations fail.
   iii. *Dorzolamide* (2%, 2-3 times/day). It is a recently introduced topical carbonic anhydrase inhibitor which lowers IOP by decreasing aqueous secretion.

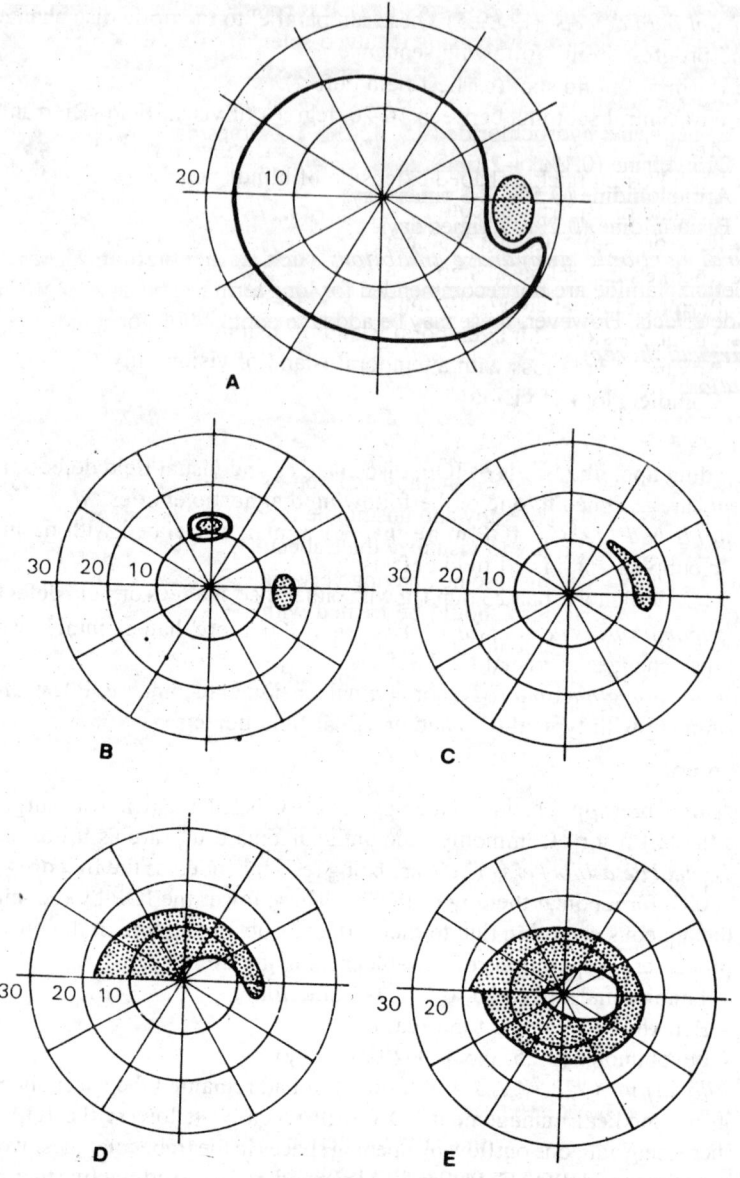

Fig. 9.5. Field defects in POAG: (A) baring of blind spot; (B) superior paracentral scotoma; (C) Seidel's scotoma; (D) Bjerrum's scotoma; (E) double arcuate scotoma and Roenne's central nasal step.

iv. *Latanoprost* (0.0005%, 2-3 times/day). It is prostaglandin by nature and decreases the IOP by increasing the uveo-scleral outflow of aqueous.

v. *Adrenergic drugs.* There are being considered as the last choice drugs. These include :
   - Epinephrine hydrochloride (0.5, 1, 2%, 1-2 times/day)
   - Dipivefrine (0.1%, 1-2 times/day)
   - Apraclonidine (0.5%, 2-3 times/day)
   - Brimonidine (0.2%, 2 times/day)

vi. *Oral carbonic anhydrase inhibitors* such as acetazolamide and methazolamide are not recommended for long term use because of their side effects. However, these may be added to control IOP for short term.

2. Surgical therapy

Indications

1. Uncontrolled glaucoma despite maximal medical therapy and laser trabeculoplasty.
2. Non-compliance of medical therapy and non-availability of ALT.
3. Failure with medical therapy and unsuitable for ALT either due to lack of cooperation or inability to visualize the trabeculum.
4. Eyes with advanced disease i.e., having very high IOP, advanced cupping and advanced field loss should be treated with filtration surgery as primary line of management.
5. Recently, some workers are even recommending surgery as primary line of treatment in all cases.

Types of surgery

Surgical treatment of POAG primarily consists of a fistulizing (filtration) surgery which provides a new channel for aqueous outflow and successfully controls the IOP (below 21 mm of Hg). Trabeculectomy is the most frequently performed filtration surgery now-a-days.

PRIMARY ANGLE CLOSURE GLAUCOMA

In it sudden rise of IOP occurs due to blockage of the aqueous outflow by closure of a narrow angle of the anterior chamber. It affects 1 in 1000 people over 40 years of age.

Etiology

(A) Predisposing factors

- Hypermetropic eyes with shallow anterior chamber.
- Eyes in which iris-lens diaphragm is placed anteriorly.
- Eyes with narrow angle of anterior chamber due to small eyeball, relative large crystalline lens, or bigger size of the ciliary body.
- Plateau iris configuration.
- Sex. Male : Female is 1 : 4

- Nervous personality with unstable vasomotor system.
- Positive family history.
- Usually fifth or sixth decade of life.

(B) *Precipitating factors*

- Dim illumination
- Emotional stress
- Use of mydriatics

(C) *Mechanism of rise in IOP*

Mid dilated pupil → increased contact between lens and iris → relative pupil block → physiological iris bombe → appositional angle closure (transient rise in IOP) → synechial angle closure → prolonged rise in IOP.

Clinical stages

1. *Prodromal stage (Latent glaucoma)*. It is characterised by intermittent attacks of transient rise in IOP associated with transient blurring of vision, coloured halos around light and mild headache.

Once clinically suspected,*diagnosis* is confirmed by prone-dark-room provocative test (positive if 8 mm of Hg pressure rise occurs in one hour).

Treatment consists of laser iridotomy or surgical peripheral iridectomy.

2. *Phase of constant instability (Intermittent or subacute glaucoma)* . Attacks of rise in IOP become more frequent and each attack lasts from few minutes to 1-2 hour.

Clinical diagnosis is confirmed by 'Prone-dark-room' provocative test.

Treatment consists of surgical peripheral iridectomy or laser iridotomy after medical control of IOP.

3. *Acute angle closure glaucoma (Acute congestive glaucoma)* : Sudden rise in IOP occurs due to total angle closure.

Symptoms are sudden onset of severe pain in the eye which radiates along the branches of 5th cranial nerve and is usually associated with nausea, vomiting and prostration, marked redness, dimness of vision, lacrimation, coloured halos (due to corneal oedema) and photophobia.

Signs : (i) Lid oedema, (ii) Marked ciliary and conjunctival congestion, (iii) corneal oedema, (iv) Mid dilated vertically oval pupil, (v) Shallow anterior chamber, (vi) Iris discolouration and stromal oedema, and (vii) Raised IOP.

Treatment

Medical

- Acetazolamide 500 mg stat and then 250 mg QID.
- Hyperosmotic agents e.g. Glycerol 1-2 g per kg body weight orally in lemon juice and/or mannitol 1-2 g per kg body weight (20% solution) given I.V. over 30 minutes.
- Pilocarpine 2-4 per cent every 15 minutes for one hour and then QID.
- Topical steroids 3-4 times a day.

- Analgesics to relieve severe pain.

Surgical
- *Peripheral iridectomy* / laser iridotomy - when peripheral anterior synechiae (PAS) are formed in less than 50 per cent of the angle of anterior chamber.
- *Filtration surgery* (e.g. Trabeculectomy) – when PAS are formed in more than 50 per cent of the angle.
- *Prophylactic* peripheral iridectomy/laser iridotomy should also be considered for the fellow eye.

4. *Chronic angle closure glaucoma* — It may develop as a sequelae to an attack of acute angle closure glaucoma or as a result of repeated subacute attacks (intermittent glaucoma) or due to gradual and progressive (creeping) synechial angle closure.

- *Clinical features*. (i) IOP remains constantly raised, (ii) Visual field defects similar to POAG are seen, (iii) Optic disc may show glaucomatous cupping, (iv) Gonioscopy reveals angle closure with peripheral anterior synechia (more marked superiorly).

- *Treatment*. Filtration surgery (trabeculectomy) should be performed after lowering the IOP by medical treatment.

5. *Absolute glaucoma* : In this end stage the eye is painful, completely blind, and IOP is very high. Cornea is clear but insensitive in early stages and may develop filamentous or bullous keratopathy in late stages. Anterior chamber is very shallow and pupil becomes fixed and dilated.

- *Complications*. Corneal ulceration, ciliary staphyloma formation and atrophic bulbi.
- *Treatment*. (i) Cyclocryotherapy, (ii) Retrobulbar injection of absolute alcohol, (iii) Enucleation for painful blind eye not responding to conservative treatment.

SECONDARY GLAUCOMAS

Raised IOP due to some other primary ocular or systemic diseases.

Classification
(A) *Depending upon the mechanism of rise in IOP*
1. *Secondary open angle glaucoma:* In these aqueous outflow may be blocked by : (a) a pretrabecular membrane (epithelial, endothelial or neovascular), (b) trabecular clogging, oedema and scarring, or (c) elevated episcleral venous pressure.
2. *Secondary angle closure glaucoma* which may or may not be associated with pupil block.

(B) *Depending upon the causative primary disease*
1. Lens induced glaucoma,

2. Inflammatory glaucoma,
3. Pigmentary glaucoma,
4. Neovascular glaucoma,
5. Pseudoexfoliative glaucoma,
6. Glaucoma associated with intraocular haemorrhages,
7. Steroid-induced glaucoma,
8. Glaucoma associated with intraocular haemorrhages,
9. Traumatic glaucoma,
10. Glaucoma in aphakia
11. Glaucoma associated with intraocular tumours.

1. Lens-induced glaucomas

- *Phacomorphic glaucoma.* IOP is raised due to secondary angle closure and/ or pupil block by lens intumescence (Pl. III.3) or, anterior subluxation or dislocation of lens or spherophakia.
- *Phacolytic glaucoma.* An acute secondary open angle glaucoma due to clogging of trabecular meshwork by macrophages laden with lens proteins in a patient with hypermature cataract.
- *Lens particle glaucoma.* It occurs due to trabecular blockage by the lens particles.
- *Phacoanaphylactic glaucoma .* It occurs due to sensitisation of eye or its fellow to lens proteins. IOP is raised due to clogging of trabeculae by inflammatory material.

2. Glaucomas due to uveitis

- *Non-specific hypertensive uveitis :* IOP is raised due to clogging by inflammatory material and associated trabeculitis.
- *Specific hypertensive uveitis syndromes :* These include : Fuch's uveitis syndrome and glaucomatocyclitic crisis.
- *Post-inflammatory glaucoma :* It may result from annular synechiae, occlusiopupillae, angle closure following iris bombe formation or angle closure due to organisation of the inflammatory debris.

3. Neovascular glaucoma

- It results due to formation of a neovascular membrane involving angle of the anterior chamber.
- Usually, stimulus to new vessel formation is retinal ischaemia as seen in diabetic retinopathy, CRVO, Eales' disease. Other rare causes are chronic uveitis, intraocular tumours, old retinal detachment, CRAO and retinopathy of prematurity.
- Neovascularisation begins at pupil and spreads centrifugally.
- Management – Panretinal photocoagulation to prevent stimulus to new vessel formation.

– Glaucoma implant (e.g. Moltena tube) operation.
– Cyclocryotherapy.

4. Glaucoma associated with intraocular tumours

. Intraocular tumours such as retinoblastoma and malignant melanoma may raise IOP by one or more of the following mechanisms :
- Trabecular block by tumour cells.
- Neovascularization of the angle.
- Venous stasis following obstruction to vortex veins.

Treatment : Enucleation of the eyeball.

5. Steroid-induced glaucoma

- Roughly, 5 per cent of general population is high steroid responder (develop marked rise of IOP after about 6 weeks of steroid therapy), 35 per cent are moderate and 60 per cent are non-responders.
- *Pathogenesis :* Probably mucopolysaccharides are deposited in the trabecular meshwork.
- Features are similar to POAG.
- *Management*
  - Can be prevented by judicious use of steroids.
  - IOP may normalise in 98 per cent of cases within 10 days to 4 weeks of discontinuation of steroids.
  - Medical therapy with 0.5% timolol maleate is effective during normalisation period.
  - Filtration surgery is required in intractable cases.

10

Diseases of Retina and Vitreous

DISEASES OF RETINA

The diseases of retina with which patient is usually hospitalized are retinal detachment and retinoblastoma. For a better nursing care the nurses need to be well conversant with these conditions. In addition certain other conditions with which a nurse should be familiar are : diabetic retinopathy, hypertensive retinopathy, retinopathy of prematurity, central retinal artery occlusion, central retinal vein occlusion and retinitis pigmentosa and solar retinopathy.

RETINAL DETACHMENT

It is the separation of retina proper (sensory retina) from the pigment epithelium. Normally these two layers are loosely attached to each other with a potential space in between. Hence actually speaking the term retinal detachment is a misnomer and it should be *retinal separation.*

Classification

1. Rhegmatogenous primary retinal detachment.
2. Secondary retinal detachment which can be :
    i. Tractional retinal detachment
    ii. Exudative retinal detachment

Etiology

I. *Primary retinal detachment*

It is usually associated with a hole or tear in the retina through which subretinal fluid (SRF) seeps and separates the sensory retina from the pigment epithelium.

Predisposing factors

1. *Age.* Most common in 40-60 years.
2. *Sex .* More common in males.
3. *Myopia* is associated in about 40 percent cases.
4. *Aphakia* is a common predisposing factor.
5. *Retinal* degenerations such as *lattice degeneration.*

6. *Trauma*
7. Senile posterior vitreous detachment (PVD).

II. *Secondary retinal detachment*

1. *Tractional retinal detachment* occurs due to pull by the fibrous tissue formation in the vitreous as seen after perforating injuries and diabetic retinopathy.
2. *Exudative retinal detachment* occurs due to the retina being pushed away from the choroid as seen in:
- Malignant melanoma of the choroid.
- Exophytic retinoblastoma.
- Haemorrhage between choroid and retina.
- Inflammations of the choroid.

Clinical features

1. *Flashes of light* (photopsia) and *dark spots* (floaters) in front of the eyes are prodromal symptoms.
2. *Localized relative loss* in the field of vision of detached retina occurs in early stages which progress gradually.
3. *Sudden painless loss of vision* occurs when the detachment is large and central. Such patients usually complain of sudden apperance of a dark cloud or curtain in front of the eye.
4. *Greyish reflex* may be seen in the pupillary area.
5. *On ophthlamoscopic examination* the detached retina gives grey reflex instead of normal pink reflex and is raised anteriorly and thrown infolds. Retina may show holes and tears.

Treatment

Usually, immediate treatment is required and patient is hospitalized.

Preoperative care

1. *Bed rest.* Patient is encouraged to complete bed rest before operation. Bed rest in a proper position (e.g. propped up position in patients with inferior retinal detachment) may prevent further separation and encourage the absorption of sub-retinal fluid.
2. *Bilateral bandage.* It is now rare for patients to have both eyes padded. Occluded glasses are more commonly worn to discourage eye movements.
3. *Atropinization.* Instillation of 1% atropine eye drops to both eyes paralyses the muscle of accommodation and provides a widely dilated pupil for the viewing of retina on indirect ophthalmoscopy.
4. *Sedatives.* During the period of waiting for surgical treatment and immobility a mild sedative may be necessary to help relieve anxiety and to control restlessness.
5. *Clinical work up.* A meticulous clinical work up including careful drawings of retina to show the position of holes and degeneration and the extent of

retinal detachment is carried out by the retinal surgeon during this waiting period.

6. *Preoperative investigation* and a full medical examination is carried out as a part of preanaesthetic check up.

7. *Social and psychological support.* In addition to an understanding and sympathetic attitude by doctors and nurses every care should be taken to meet patient's social and psychological need by the friends and family members.

Surgical treatment

Basic principles of surgical treatment are as follows:

1. *Sealing of retinal breaks.* All the retinal breaks should be detected, accurately localised and sealed by producing aseptic chorioretinitis, with cryocoagulation, photocoagulation or diathermy. Cryocoagulation is more frequently utilised (Fig. 10.1).

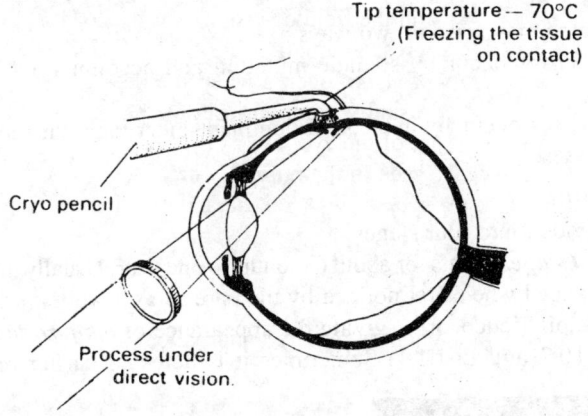

Fig. 10.1. Cryocoagulation of the retinal hole area under direct vision with indirect ophthalmoscopy.

2. *To bring the sclerochoroid and detached retina near to each other.* This is carried out by the procedure of *scleral buckling or encirclage* . In addition, any of the following procedures may also be required:

   i. *Drainage* of SRF is required in long-standing cases.

   ii. *Internal tamponade* by SF_6 gas or silicone oil is required in complicated cases.

   iii. *Pars plana vitrectomy* is required to cut the vitreoretinal tractional bands.

Postoperative nursing care

1. *Immediate postoperative nursing care* is in the way usual for all patients following general anaesthesia (see page 42).
2. *Postoperative nursing care* during patients stage in the hospital is similar to that for a patient after a cataract extraction (see page 42-44).

Instructions at discharge

1. Patient should be advised to avoid straining of any kind and heavy lifting and should perform only light tasks for 3-4 weeks postoperatively.
2. If patient's profession involves heavy manual labour he may be advised to look for some lighter alternative work to earn livelihood.

RETINOBLASTOMA

It is a common congenital malignant tumour of retina. Though usually congenital, it is not recognised at birth and is usually seen between 1-2 years of age. It may be unilateral or bilateral (20-30 percent cases).

Etiology

Retinoblastoma may arise in two ways :

1. *Sporadic cases* occur by somatic mutation and account for 94 percent cases.
2. Familial cases occur by autosomal dominant inheritance in remaining 6 percent cases.

Clinical picture

It may be divided into four stages :

1. *Quiescent stage.* It lasts for about 6 months to one year. Usually the tumour is fairly advanced when first noticed by the parents as a white mass behind the dilated pupil (leucocoria) giving the appearance of *amaurotic cat's eye reflex.* (Fig.10.2 and Pl III.4) Sometimes it is detected earlier on fundus

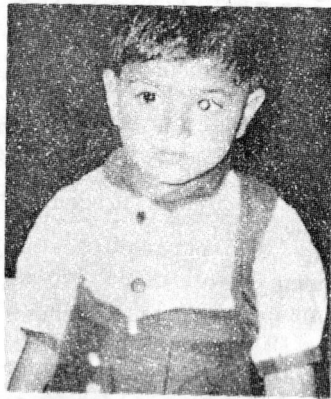

Fig. 10.2. Leukocoria left eye in a patient with retinoblastoma

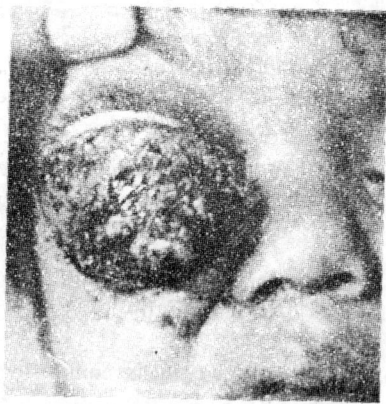

Fig. 10.3. Fungating retinoblastoma involving the orbit.

examination if the infant or child is brought with squint which arises as a result of loss of vision in the affected eye.

2. Glaucomatous stage. It develops when retinoblastoma is left untreated during quiescent stage. This stage is characterized by severe pain, redness, watering and hazy cornea due to raised intraocular pressure.

3. Stage of extraocular extension. Due to progressive enlargement, the globe bursts through the sclera, usually at the limbus. It is followed by rapid fungation and involvement of extraocular tissues resulting in marked proptosis (Fig.10.3).

4. Stage of distant metastasis. Metastasis may occur by :
 – Lymphatic spread in the preauricular and neighbouring lymph nodes.
 – *Direct extension* to the optic nerve and brain.
 – *Blood spread* to cranial and other bones and rarely to other organs.

Treatment

1. *In early stages* (when tumour is less than 10 mm) treatment can be carried out successfully by the application of *radioactive cobalt plaques* over the site of growth. For small tumour located posteriorly, *photocogulation* may be useful.
2. *In advanced cases* the treatment of choice is *enucleation* (removal) of the affected eyeball, together with as much of the optic nerve as possible.

Nursing care

1. *Handling of parents.* Role of a nurse in case of a child admitted for enucleation is not only limited to care of the child but also to care for the emotional and mental preparation and counselling of the parents.
2. *Preoperative care* is similar to that of a child for any surgery under general anaesthesia (see page 41).
3. *Postoperative general nursing care* of child has also been described earlier (see page 42-44).
4. *Postoperative ocular nursing care* after enucleation operation includes regular gentle cleansing of the eye and fitting of the conformer/glass shell for first two weeks. It is followed by fitting of an artificial eye. Child may accept the fitting of a shell well, but much patience and fact may be needed when instructing the parents in the care of the shell as they find the procedure unpleasant and difficult to accept.
5. *Instructions during discharge.* In addition to the proper care of artificial eye, the parents should be instructed about the need for frequent follow ups to detect any recurrence or involvement of the other eye at an early stage. The parents should also be advised that their other children should also be examined in order to exclude the presence of tumour in their eyes. The genetic counselling should also be discussed with the parents.

CENTRAL RETINAL ARTERY OCCLUSION

Central retinal artery occlusion (CRAO) may occur due to embolus, thrombosis or arteritis. It is more common in patients suffering from hypertension and other cardiovascular diseases.

CRAO is characterized by a sudden and total painless loss of vision which unfortunately is usually irreversible, since retina can survive ischaemia only for an hour or so and by the time patient is examined, it is too late.

CENTRAL RETINAL VEIN OCCLUSION

Central retinal vein occlusion (CRVO) is more common than the artery occlusion. It is usually associated with arterio-sclerotic changes. It is characterized by a sudden but incomplete loss of vision associated with multiple retinal haemorrhages usually, self-recovery occurs and so no treatment is required. In few cases of ischaemia CRVO, neovascularization occurs which may be complicated by *neovascular glaucoma.* This catastrophe may be prevented by timely panretinal photocoagulation (PRP).

DIABETIC RETINOPATHY

Diabetic retinopathy refers to the retinal changes seen in patients with diabetes mellitus. With increase in the life expectancy of diabetics, the incidence of diabetic retinopathy has increased. Duration of diabetes is the most important determining factors.

Clinical features

Clinically diabetic retinopathy can be classified into following types :
1. *Background diabetic retinopathy (BDR).* Retinal changes in BDR are capillary microaneurysms, retinal haemorrhages, hard exudates and retinal oedema.
2. *Diabetic maculopathy* refers to involvement of macular area by the above changes.
3. *Pre-proliferative diabetic retinopathy* consists of changes of acute retinal ischaemia superadded over the changes of BDR. These include cotton-wool patches, intra-retinal microvascular abnormolities (IRMA), venous dilatation and beading and large dark blot haemorrhage.
4. *Proliferative diabetic retinopathy (PDR)* is characterized by occurrence of neovascularization over the changes of pre-proliferative diabetic retinopathy.
5. *Advanced diabetic eye disease* is the end - result of uncontrolled PDR. It is marked by complications such as vitreous haemorrhage, tractional retinal detachment and neovascular glaucoma.

Management

1. **Strict control** of blood glucose may delay the onset and reduce the severity of retinopathy.

2. A regular periodic follow up is of utmost importance for timely intervention.

3. *Photocoagulation* is indicated as below :
   - *Panretinal photocoagulation* (PRP) is indicated in patients with PDR with one of the high risk characteristics (HRC).
   - *Focal argon laser burns* are useful in patients with focal exudative maculopathy.
   - *Grid pattern laser burns* are applied in macular area for diffuse macular oedema.
   - *Surgical treatment* is indicated in patients with dense persistent vitreous haemorrhage and tractional retinal detachment.

HYPERTENSIVE RETINOPATHY

Hypertensive retinopathy refers to fundus changes occurring in patients suffering from systemic hypertension. It has been classified into four grades I to IV. They reflect the severity and duration of hypertension.

RETINOPATHY OF PREMATURITY

Retinopathy of prematurity (old name : Retrolental fibroplasia) refers to bilateral proliferative retinopathy occuring in premature infants (weighing less than 1300 gm) exposed to high concentration of oxygen during first 10 days of life. Therefore, staff nurse especially these posted in paediatric nurseries must be aware of this condition. Depending upon the severity of retinoproliferative changes the ROP has been divided into 5 stages (1 to 5).

Treatment in advanced stage (4 and 5) is frustrating. So a prophylaxis and regular screening of such infants every week is of utmost importance for a timely intervention by lasers or cryo application.

RETINITIS PIGMENTOSA

Retinitis pigmentosa (RP) is a hereditary primary pigment dystrophy affecting the rods more than the cones. Most common mode of inheritance is autosomal recessive. Night blindness is its characteristic feature and occurs several years before the visible changes in the retina appear. The onset is after teens with gross handicap occurring in middle or adnormal age. Retinal pigmentary changes are typically perivascular and resemble *bone corpuscles* in shape. Initially the changes are found in the equatorial region only and later spread both anteriorly and posteriorly. Retinal arterioles are attenuated (narrowed) and may become thread-like in late stages. Eventually consecutive optic atrophy sets in.

In early stages the disease is confirmed by occurrence of typical electroretinographic (ERG) changes which appear much before the fundus changes.

No effective treatment is available for the disease. Low vision aids (LVA) may be of some help untill blindness is total.

DISEASES OF THE VITREOUS

VITREOUS OPACITIES

Normal vitreous is a transparent structure. Therefore, any relatively non-transparent structure present in it will form an opacity. *Common causes* of vitreous opacities are as follows :

1. *Development opacities* are seen rarely and represent the remnants of the hyaloid vasculature. *Persistent hyperplastic primary vitreous (PHPV)* which results from failure of the primary vitreous structure to develop is clinically characterized by a white pupillary reflex (leucocoria)
2. *Inflammatory opacities* consist of exudates in the vitreous seen is patients with inflammation of uveal tissue and retina.
3. *Amyloid degeneration* is a rare condition in which amorphous amyloid material is deposited in the vitreous.
4. *Asteroid hyalosis* is characterized by small rounded bodies suspended in the vitreous gel. It is usually seen in one eye of the elderly people.
5. *Synchysis scintillans* refers to small white angular and crystalline bodies formed of cholesterol seen in eyes which have suffered in the part by trauma or inflammation.

VITREOUS DETACHMENT

Normally vitreous is attached with retina, pars plana, part of ciliary body and back of lens. Strongest attachment is in the area of *vitreous base* (4 mm wide area of attachment to the ora serrata). Following types of vitreous detachments may occur.

1. *Posterior vitreous detachment (PVD)* i.e. detachment of vitreous from retina posterior to vitreous base. PVD is of common occurrence in majority of the normal subjects above the age of 65 years. It may be associated with flashes of light and floaters in front of the eyes.
2. *Anterior and basal vitreous detachment* usually occur secondary to blunt trauma and may be associated with anterior retinal dialysis, dislocation of lens and vitreous haemorrhage.

VITREOUS HAEMORRHAGE

Vitreous haemorrhage usually occurs from the retinal vessels. It presents with sudden onset of floaters to significant loss of vision. Its common causes are :

1. Spontaneous retinal breaks associated with PVD.
2. Trauma to eye.
3. Proliferative retinopathies such as diabetic retinopathy, Eales' disease, and sickle cell retinopathy.

11

Squint and Nystagmus

SQUINT

Normally visual axes of the two eyes are parallel to each other in the primary position of gaze and this alignment is maintained in all the positions except in convergence and divergence.

A misalignment of the visual axes of the two eyes is called squint or strabismus.

Types and Etiology

Broadly squint is of following types :

1. Latent squint (Heterophoria). In this condition the tendency of the two eyes to deviate is kept latent by the faculty of fusion. Therefore, when the influence of fusion is removed e.g. when one eye is covered this will deviate away. Common types are esophoria and exophoria.

2. Manifest squint (Heterotropia). It is manifest deviation of the eye under binocular conditions. It is mainly of two types :

i. *Concomitant squint*. Here in the amount of deviation in the squinting eye remains constant in all the direction of gaze. Common causes of concomitant squint are refractive errors, abnormalities of accommodations, convergence and AC/A ratio, unilateral loss of vision and heredity. It can be classified in different ways as follows :

a) Depending upon the direction of deviations

- *Esotropia* or *convergent squint* i.e. inward deviation of the globe.
- *Exotropia or divergent squint* i.e. outward deviation of the eyeball.
- *Hypertropia or vertical squint* i.e. one eye is placed upwards as compared to the other.

b) Depending upon the fixation behaviour

- *Uniocular squint* i.e. the same one eye always deviates and the second normal eye takes fixation.
- *Alternate squint* i.e. either of the eye can deviate and the other eye will take fixation.

c) Depending upon the constancy of deviation
- *Constant squint* i.e. when the squint is present all the times.
- Intermittent squint .

ii. *Paralytic squint.* It is type of incomitant squint i.e. in which the amount of deviation varies in different directions of gaze. It results from complete or incomplete paralysis of one or more extraocular muscles.

Common causes of paralytic squint. Paralytic squint may occur due to lesions of nerve or muscles. Common causes are :

1. *Inflammation* in the form of neuritis or myositis.
2. *Vascular lesions* like haemorrhage, thrombosis, embolism, aneurysm.
3. *Traumatic lesions*
4. *Metabolic* disorders like diabetes mellitus.
5. *Tumours,* such as brain tumours involving nuclei nerve roots or intracranial part of nerves.
6. *Demyelinating* lesions like multiple sclerosis.

Clinical features

1. *Deviation* of the eyeball depending upon the type i.e. convergent (Fig. 11.1), divergent (Fig. 11.2) or vertical.

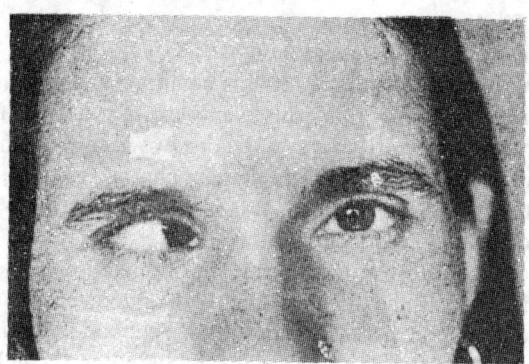

Fig. 11.1. Concomitant squint, (right) esotropia.

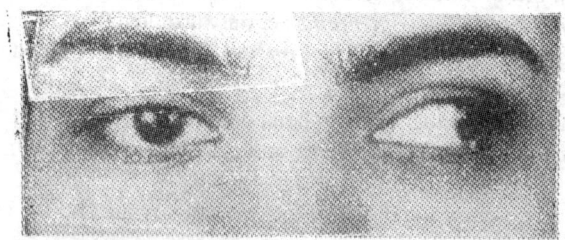

Fig. 11.2. A patient with primary exotropia.

2. *Movements* of eyeball are defective in paralytic squint.
3. *Diplopia* and abnormal head posture are features of paralytic squint.

Trea⁺ment

1. *Optical correction of refractive error* is the first step in the management of squint.
2. *Occlusion therapy* is required to treat associated amblyopia. Normal eye should be occluded to force the child to use amblyopic eye.
3. *Orthoptic exercises* with synoptophore are given to overcome the suppression, to improve convergence insufficiency and to improve fusion range.
4. *Squint surgery* is required in most cases to correct the deviation. Common operations are :
   i. *Resection.* In this procedure the extraocular muscle is strengthened by shortening its effective length.
   ii. *Recession.* In this procedure the extraocular muscle is weakened by shifting its insertion posteriorly.

Nursing care in squint surgery

1. Preoperative nursing care for operation under general anaesthesia (see page 41).
2. Antibiotic drops are to be instilled preoperatively.
3. Postoperative general care after operation under general anaesthesia (see page 42-44).
4. The eye is bandaged for one day only. From second day topical antibiotic drops are to be used and the eye is kept open.
5. The eye will be red and this will cause the mother to be concerned; she should be reassured that the redness of the eye will subside in two to three weeks.

NYSTAGMUS

It is defined as regular and rhythmic to-and-fro involuntary oscillatory movements of the eyes.

Types and etiology

1. *Physiological nystagmus* e.g. optokinetic nystagmus (OKN).
2. *Sensory deprivations (ocular)* nystagmus. It may be congenital or acquired.
3. *Motor imbalance nystagmus* e.g. congenital jerk nystagmus.

Clinical features

1. It may be pendular or jerk nystagmus.
2. Nystagmus may be vertical, horizontal or rotatory.
3. Nystagmus movements may be rapid or slow.
4. The movements of eye may be fine or coarse.
5. Nystagmus may be latent or manifest.

12

Neuro-ophthalmology

LESIONS OF VISUAL PATHWAY

Visual disturbances produced by the lesion at different levels of visual pathway are as follows (Fig.12.1).

1. *Lesions of the optic nerve* produce marked loss of vision or complete blindness on the affected side.
2. *Centrol lesion of the optic chiasma* produce bitemporal hemianopia.
3. *Lateral chiasmal lesions* produce binasal hemianopia.
4. *Lesions of optic tract, lateral geniculate body and visual cortex* produce homonymous hemianopia.

PUPILLARY REFLEX AND THEIR ABNORMALITIES

Light reflex

When light is shown in one eye, both the pupils constrict. Constriction of the pupil to which light is shown is called *direct light reflex* and that of the other pupil is called *consensual (indirect) light reflex.*

Light reflex is initiated by rods and cones. Afferent fibres travel along the optic nerve upto lateral geniculate body and terminate in the Edinger-Westphal nucleus from where efferent parasympathetic fibres start and travel along the oculomotor nerve. These ultimately reach the sphincter pupillae muscle (Fig. 12.2).

Near reflex

Near reflex occurs on looking at a near object. It consists of two components: (a) convergence reflex i.e. contraction of pupil on convergence; and (b) accommodation reflex i.e. contraction of pupil associated with accommodation.

ABNORMALITIES OF PUPILLARY REACTIONS

1. Amaurotic light reflex. It reters to the absence of direct light reflex on the affected side (say right eye) and absence of consensual light reflex on the

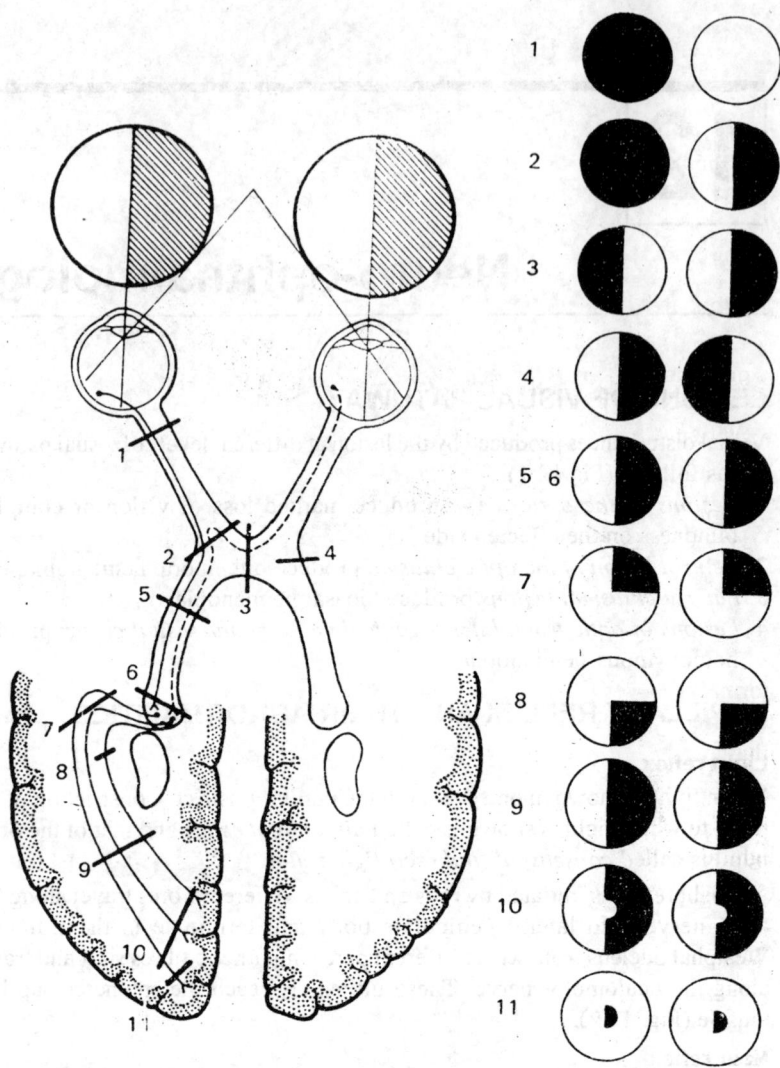

Fig. 12.1. Lesions of the visual pathways at the level of: 1. optic nerve; 2. proximal part of optic nerve; 3. central chiasma; 4. lateral chiasma (both sides); 5. optic tract; 6. geniculate body; 7. part of optic radiations in temporal lobe; 8. part of optic radiations in parietal lobe; 9. optic radiations; 10. visual cortex sparing the macula; 11. visual cortex, only macula.

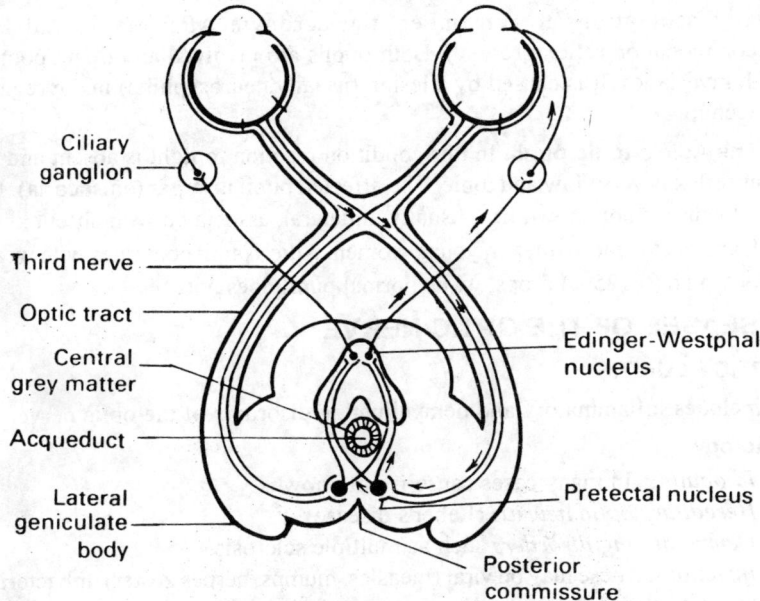

Fig. 12.2. Pathway of the light reflex.

normal side (i.e. left eye). This indicates lesions of the optic nerve or retina on the affected side (i.e. right eye), leading to complete blindness. In diffuse illumination both pupils are of equal size.

2. Efferent pathway defect. Absence of both direct and consensual light reflex on the affected side (say right eye) and presence of both direct and consensual light reflex on the normal side (i.e. left eye) indicates efferent pathway defect (sphincter paralysis). Near reflex is also absent on the affected side. Its causes include: effect of parasympatholytic drugs (e.g. atropine, homatropine), internal ophthalmoplegia, and third nerve paralysis.

3. Wernicke's hemianopic pupil. It indicates lesion of the optic tract. In this condition light reflex (ipsilateral direct and contralateral consensual) is absent when light is thrown on the temporal half of the retina of the affected side and nasal half of the opposite side; while it is present when the light is thrown on the nasal half of the affected side and temporal half of the opposite side.

4. Marcus Gunn pupil . It is the paradoxical response of a pupil of light in the presence of a relative afferent pathway defect (RAPD). It is tested by swinging flash light test.

5. Argyll Robertson pupil (ARP). Here the pupil is slightly small in size and reaction to near reflex is present but light reflex is absent, i.e., there is light near dissociation (to remember, the acronym ARP may stand for 'accommodation reflex present'). Both pupils are involved and dilate poorly with mydriatics. It is caused by a lesion (usually neurosyphilis) in the region of tectum.٭

6. The Adie's tonic pupil. In this condition reaction to light is absent and to near reflex is very slow and tonic. The affected pupil is larger (anisocoria). Its exact cause is not known. It is usually unilateral, associated with absent knee jerk and occurs more often in young women. Adie's pupil constricts with weak pilocarpine (0.125%) drops, while normal pupil does not.

DISEASES OF THE OPTIC NERVE

OPTIC NEURITIS

It includes inflammatory and demyelinating disorders of the optic nerve.

Etiology

1. *Idiopathic.* In many cases cause is not known.
2. *Hereditary optic neuritis* (Leber's disease)
3. *Demyelinating disorders* such as multiple sclerosis.
4. *Infections.* These may be viral (measles, mumps, herpes zoster) or bacterial (e.g. as seen in meningococcal meningitis)
5. *Toxic optic neuritis* occurs due to the effects of exogenous or endogenous poisons.

Clinical types

1. *Papillitis.* It is the acute inflammation of optic disc. It is characterized by sudden and profound loss of vision. Ophthalmoscopic examination reveals hyperaemia and oedema of the disc with blurring of its margins.
2. *Acute retrobulbar neuritis.* It is an acute inflammation of the optic nerve behind the eyeball. It is characterized by sudden and profound loss of vision but fundus examination is normal.
3. *Toxic amblyopias.* These include chronic retrobulbar neuritis occuring due to effect of various toxins. Common conditions are tobacco amblyopia, ethyl alcohol amblyopia, quinine amblyopia and ethambutol amblyopia.

PAPILLOEDEMA

The term papilloedema has been reserved for the passive disc swelling associated with increased intracranial pressure.

Etiology

1. *Congenital conditions* include aqueductal stenosis and cranio-synostosis.
2. *Intracranial space-occupying lesions* (ICSOLs) such as brain tumours, subdural haematomas and aneurysm. ICSOLs are common causes of papilloedema.
3. *Intracranial infections* suchs as encephalitis and meningitis.

4. *Intracranial haemorrhage* e.g. subarachnoid haemorrhage.
5. *Tumours of spinal cord*
6. *Pseudotumour cerebri* i.e. benign raised intracranial pressure.

Clinical features

1. *General features* of raised intracranial pressure include headache, nausea, vomiting and diplopia.
2. *Ocular features.* Usually vision is normal but patient may give history of transient blackouts. On ophthalmoscopic examination papilloedema is characterized by hyperaemia and marked swelling of the optic disc with blurring of its margins. Papilloedema is usually bilateral. In long-standing cases optic atrophy sets in and vision is lost.

Treatment

It is a neurological emergency and requires immediate hospitalization and management by neurosurgeon.
Nursing care is that of a critically ill patient.

OPTIC ATROPHY

Optic atrophy is the degeneration of optic nerve fibres. It is characterized by pallor of the optic disc. Optic atrophy is of following types.

1. *Primary optic atrophy* occurs in patients with multiple sclerosis, tabes dorsalis and Leber's hereditary optic atrophy.
2. *Consecutive optic atrophy* occurs secondary to certain retinal diseases such as retinitis pigmentosa and extensive retinochoroiditis.
3. *Postneuritic optic atrophy* develops as a sequel to long-standing papillitis or papilloedema.
4. *Glaucomatous optic atrophy* results due to damage to retinal nerve fibres by raised intraocular pressure.
5. *I schhaemic optic atrophy* is seen in patients with giant cell arteritis.

SYMPTOMATIC DISTURBANCES OF VISION

NIGHT BLINDNESS (Nyctalopia)

Night (scotopic) vision is a function of rod cells of the retina. Therefore, the conditions in which functioning of the rod cells is deranged will result in night blindness. The most common causes of night blindness are vitamin A deficiency and retinitis pigmentosa.

DAY BLINDNESS (Hamarlopia)

It is a symptomatic disturbance of the vision, in which the patient is able to see better in dimlight as compared to bright light of the day. Its causes are congenital deficiency of cones, central lenticular opacities (polar cataracts) and central corneal opacities.

COLOUR BLINDNESS

Normal colour vision is trichromatic i.e. we can recognise the three primary colours (red, green and blue) and their combinations. In colour blindness faculty to appreciate one or more primary colours is either defective (anomalous) or absent (anopia). It may be *congenital* (more common) or *acquired.* Depending on the type and degree of primary colour deficieny the colour blindness is of following types:

- Protanamalous – Partial red colour deficiency
- Protanopia – Complete red colour deficiency
- Deuteranomalous – Partial green colour deficiency
- Deuteranopia – Complete red colour deficiency
- Tritanamalous – Partial blue colour deficiency
- Tritanopia – Complete blue colour deficiency
- Achromatopsia – Total colour blindness (all the three primary colours are absent).

AMAUROSIS

Amaurosis refers to sudden and total loss of sight in one or both eyes, in the absence of ophthalmoscopic or other marked objective signs. *Amaurosis fugax* is the term used to describe temporary, painless monocular visual loss occuring due to a transient failure of retinal circulation seen in patients with cardio-vascular disorders.

AMBLYOPIA

Amblyopia refers to partial loss of sight in one or both eyes, in the absence of ophthalmoscopic or other marked objective signs. Functional amblyopia results from the psychical suppression of the retinal image. Depending upon the etiology it is of following types:

- Anisometropic amblyopia
- Strabismic amblyopia
- Stimulus deprivation amblyopia

MALINGERING BLINDNESS

In it a person poses to be visually defective, while he is not. The person may do so to gain some advantage of compensation. Usually one eye is said to be blind which does not show any objective sign. *Malingering needs to be established by careful examination by the ophthalmologist.*

HYSTERICAL BLINDNESS

It is a form of psychoneurosis, commonly seen in attention-seeking personalities, especially females. It is characterized by sudden bilateral loss of vision (cf. malingering). The patient otherwise shows little concern for the symptoms and negotiates well with the surroundings (cf. malingering).

13

Diseases of the Eyelids

CONGENITAL ANOMALIES

A few congenital anomalies with which a nurse need to be familiar are as follows :

1. **Congenital ptosis.** It is the most common congenital anomaly. It is described in detail under the section of ptosis.

2. **Congenital coloboma.** It is a rare condition characterized by a full thickness triangular gap in the tissues of the eyelids.

3. **Epicanthus.** It refers to a semicircular fold of skin which covers the medial canthus. It is a bilateral condition and may disappear with the development of face. It is a normal facial feature in mongolian races.

4. **Districhiasis.** It is a rare anomaly in which an extra row of cilia occupies the position of Meibomian glands. These cilia are usually directed backwards and rub the cornea. These need to be electroepilated.

INFLAMMATORY DISORDERS

BLEPHARITIS

It is an extremely common, chronic inflammation of the lid margin. Its two common forms are squamous and ulcerative blepharitis.

Squamous or seborrhoeic blepharitis

Etiology. It is usually associated with seborrhoea of the scalp (dandruf). Some metabolic and constitutional factors play a part in its etiology.

Clinical features. It is characterized by redness and swelling of the lid margin associated with deposition of white scale like dandruf material. Patient feels discomfort and irritation. On removing the scales underlying surface is found to be hyperaemic (no ulcers). The lashes fall out frequently.

Treatment. Scales should be removed with the help of a baby shampoo followed by frequent application of combined antibiotic and steroid eye ointment.

Ulcerative Blepharitis

Etiology. It is a chronic staphylococcal infection of the lid margin. Poor hygienic conditions, eye strain, chronic conjunctivitis and chronic nasal infection are common predisposing factors.

Clinical features. It is characterised by *yellow crust* formation at the root of cilia which glue them together (Fig. 13.1). Small *ulcers* which bleed easily are seen on removing the crusts. Patients often experience irritation, lacrimation and photophobia.

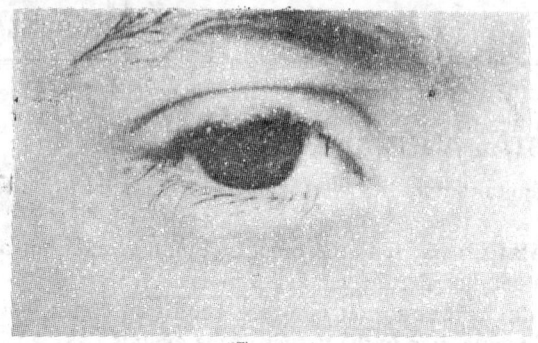

Fig. 13.1. Ulcerative blepharitis.

Treatment

1. *General health hygiene* and nutrition of the child should be improved.
2. *Crusts* should be removed after softening and hot compresses with 3% soda bicarb solution.
3. *Antibiotic ointment* should be applied 3-4 times a day.

STYE (HORDEOLUM EXTERNUM)

It is an acute suppurative inflammation of the Zeis gland and eyelash follicles.

Etiology

It is a staphylococcal infection occurring more commonly in children and young adults. Common predisposing factors are eye strain, habitual rubbing of the eyes, chronic blepharitis, diabetes mellitus and chronic debility.

Clinical features

It is characterized by a painful swelling at the lid margin associated with lid oedema (Pl. III.5) mild watering and photophobia. In advanced cases a pus point is visible on the lid margin in relation to the involved cilia.

Treatment

1. *Hot compresses* with moist heat 2-3 times a day are very useful.
2. *Evacuation of pus* by epilating the involved cilia should be carried out when pus point is formed.
3. *Antibiotics* eye drops (3-4 times a day) and ointment at night should be applied.

4. *Systemic antibiotics* may be used for early control of infection.
5. *Analgesics* may be required to relieve the pain.
6. *In recurrent cases* efforts should be made to find out and eliminate the predisposing factor. Proper ocular hygiene is very important.

CHALAZION

It is a chronic non-infective granulomatous inflammation of the meibomian glands of the eyelids.

Etiology

Predisposing factors are similar to that described for stye. Intially there occurs blockage of the duct of meibomian gland followed by retention of secretions (sebum) in the gland, causing its enlargement. The pentup secretions (fatty in nature) act like an irritant and excite non-infective granulomatous inflammation of the meibomian gland.

Clinical picture

Patient usually presents with a painless swelling in the lid which is firm to hard, non-tender, present slightly away from the lid margin (Fig.13.2). It usually points on the conjunctival side. Frequently more than one chalazion may be seen involving more than one eye lid. When infected it becomes very painful and the condition is known as *hordeolum internum.*

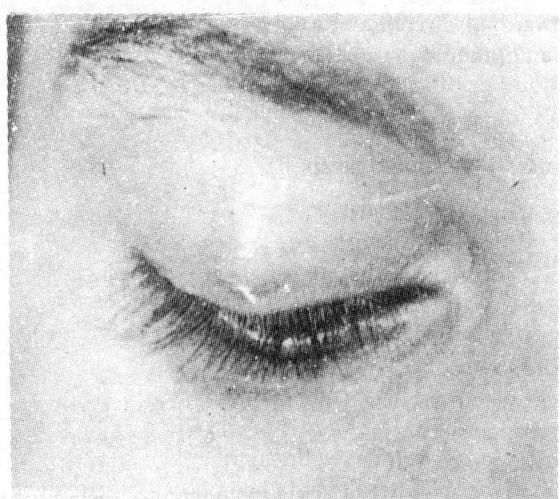

Fig. 13.2. Chalazion right upper lid.

Treatment

1. *Conservative treatment* in the form of hot fomentation, antibiotics and anti-inflammatory drugs may be useful in small, soft and recent chalazia.

2. *Intralesional injection* of long-acting steroids (triamcinolone) is also helpful in fresh chalazion.
3. *Incision and curretage* from the conjunctival side (Fig. 13.3) is the conventional and most effective treatment for chalazion. Post-operatively, hot fomentation, antibiotics and anti-inflammatory drugs are required.

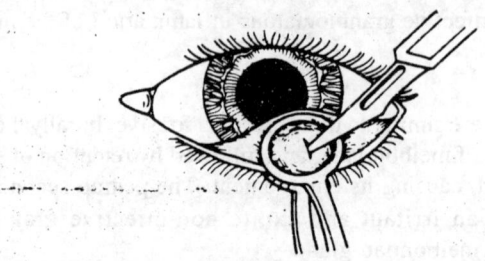

Fig. 13.3. Incision and curretage of chalazion from the conjunctival side.

ANOMALIES IN THE POSITION OF THE LASHES AND LID MARGIN

TRICHIASIS

It refers to inward misdirection of cilia (which rub against the cornea) with normal position of the lid margin (Fig.13.4).

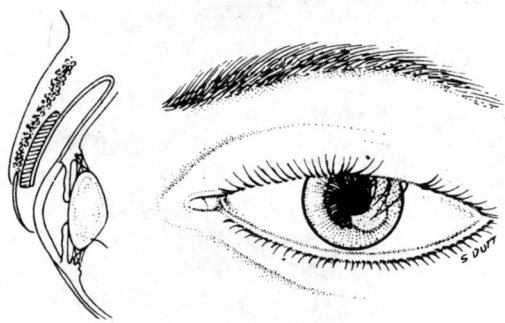

Fig. 13.4. Trichiasis.

Etiology. Common causes of trichiasis are trachoma, ulcerative blepharitis, burns and injuries of the lid margin.

Clinical features. The misdirected cilia rub against the eyeball and lead on to foreign body sensation, photophobia, pain and lacrimation.

Treatment. When many cilia are misdirected operative treatment is similar to that described for cicatricial entropion. A few misdirected cilia may be treated by any of the following methods :

1. *Epilation* (mechanical removal with forceps). It is a temporary method, as recurrence occurs within 3-4 weeks.
2. *Electrolysis.* It is method of destroying the lash follicles permanently by electric current of 2 mA passed for 10 seconds.
3. *Cryoepilation.* It is a method of destroying lash follicle permanently by freezing them ($-20°C$) with cryoprobe.

ENTROPION

It refers to inturning of the eyelid margin.

Types and etiology

1. *Congenital entropion.* It is rare congenital anomaly seen since birth.
2. *Cicatricial entropion.* It is caused by scarring of the palpebral conjunctiva. It is more common in upper eyelid. Common causes are trachoma, membranous conjunctivitis and chemical burns.
3. *Senile entropion.* It occurs in elderly people in the lower eyelids due to atrophy of the supporting tissues.
4. *Mechanical entropion.* It occurs due to lack of support provided by the eyeball. Therefore, it is seen in patients with phthisis bulbi and those in which eyeball has been removed.

Clinical picture

Symptoms occurs due to rubbing of cilia against the cornea and conjunctiva and are thus similar to trichiasis. These include foreign body sensation, irritation, lacrimation and photophobia.
Signs. On examination the margin of eyelid is found inturned.
Treatment. Surgical correction is needed depending upon the cause.

1. *Cicatricial entropion* is corrected by any of the following operations.
   - Tarsal wedge resection operation
   - Modified Ketssey's operations
2. *Senile entropion.* Common operations are:
   - Modified Wheeler's operation, in which double breasting of orbicularis oculi muscle is done.
   - Tucking or plication of inferior lid retractors is useful in severe cases.

ECTROPION

Outward turning of the lid margin is called ectropion.

Types and etiology

1. *Senile ectropion.* It is the commonest variety and involves only the lower lids. It occurs due to laxity of the tissues of the lids and loss of tone of the orbicularis muscle in old age.
2. *Cicatricial ectropion.* It occurs due to scarring of the skin of lids (Fig. 13.5) after trauma, burns and ulcers.

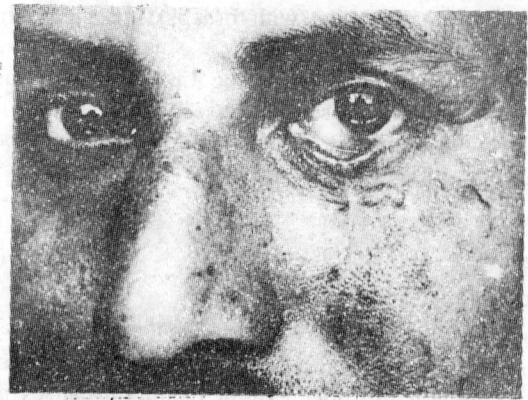

Fig. 13.5. Cicatricial ectropion left lower lid.

3. *Paralytic ectropion.* It results due to paralysis of seventh nerve which supplies the orbicularis oculi muscle. Common causes of facial nerve paralysis are Bell's palsy, head injury and infections of the middle ear.

4. *Mechanical ectropion.* It occurs due to tumours which pull the lower lid down.

Clinical picture

1. *Epiphora (watering from the eye)* is the main symptom.
2. *Out turning* of the lid margin is observed on examination.
3. *Signs of causative condition* such as skin scarring, paralysis of 7th nerve etc may be seen.

Treatment

Surgical correction is needed, depending upon the cause of ectropion.

PTOSIS

Abnormal drooping of the upper eyelid is called ptosis. Normally, upper lid covers about upper one-sixth of the cornea, i.e. about 2 mm. Therefore, in ptosis, it covers more than 2 mm.

Types and etiology

I. *Congenital ptosis.* It is associated with congenital weakness of the levator palpebrae superior is muscle.

II. *Acquired ptosis.* Depending upon the cause it can be of following types :

1. *Neurogenic ptosis.* It is caused by paralysis of the levator or Muller's muscle of the upper lid.
2. *Senile ptosis.* It is seen in old age.
3. *Traumatic ptosis.* Follows trauma to the upper lid.
4. *Mechanical ptosis* occurs due to excessive weight on the upper lid as seen in patients with tumours of the upper lid.
5. *Myogenic ptosis* is seen in patients with myasthaenia gravis.

Clinical picture

1. *Palpebral aperture* of the involved eye is small due to drooping of the upper eyelid, so the eye looks small (Fig. 13.6).
2. Vision may be obstructed if the upper lid covers the pupil.
3. Patient may try to open the eyes forcibly especially in bilateral cases leading to wrinkles on the forehead.

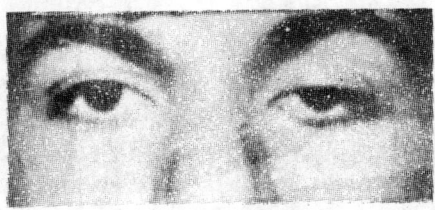

Fig. 13.6. Congenital ptosis.

Treatment

Ptosis is corrected by surgery depending upon the degree of ptosis and amount of levator function. Common operation are levator resection, Mullerotarsectomy and frontalis sling operation.

TUMOURS OF THE EYELIDS

Common tumours which can involve the lids are as follows :

1. *Benign tumours.* These include papilloma, haemangioma and neurofibroma.
2. *Malignant tumours.* These include squamous cell carcinoma, basal cell carcinoma, malignant melanoma and sebaceous gland carcinoma.

14

Diseases of the Lacrimal Apparatus

TEAR FILM AND ITS ABNORMALITIES

TEAR FILM

Tear film refers to the fluid covering the cornea and conjunctiva. Tears are composed of 98% water and 1.5% sodium chloride (which gives to the tears their salty flavour). It also contains antibacterial substances like lysozyme, betalysin and lactoferrin. Anatomically the precorneal tear film has been described to consist of three layers, which from posterior to anterior (Fig.14.1) are :

1. *Mucin layer.* It consists of mucus secreted by conjunctival goblet cells.
2. *Aqueous layer.* It is formed by the tears secreted by the main and accessory lacrimal glands.
3. *Lipid layer.* This, outermost layer, is formed by secretions of Meibomian, Zeis and Moll glands.

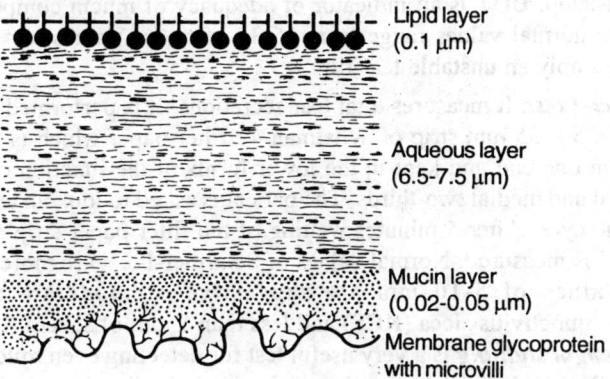

Lipid layer
(0.1 µm)

Aqueous layer
(6.5-7.5 µm)

Mucin layer
(0.02-0.05 µm)

Membrane glycoprotein
with microvilli

Fig. 14.1. Structure of the tear film.

DRY EYE

Dry eye per se is not a disease entity, but a symptom complex occurring as a sequelae to deficiency or abnormalities of tear film.

Etiology

1. *Sjogren's disease* is the most common cause of aqueous tear deficiency (*keratoconjunctivitis sicca*). It is an autoimmune chronic inflammatory disease particularly affecting lacrimal and salivary glands. Therefore, patients have dry eye and dry mouth. It is seen more commonly in women between 40-50 years. Rheumatoid arthritis is a common association.
2. *Conjunctival scarring diseases* such as trachoma, chemical burns and ocular pemphigoid are also common causes of dry eye.
3. *Lid diseases* such as chronic blepharitis and ectropion may also lead to dry eye condition.

Clinical features

Symptoms suggestive of dry eye include irritation, foreign body (sandy) sensation, feeling of dryness, itching, non-specific ocular discomfort and chronically sore eyes not responding to a variety of drops instilled earlier.

Signs of dry eye include : presence of stringy mucus and particulate matter in the tear film, lustreless ocular surface, conjunctival xerosis, Bitot spots, reduced or absent marginal tear strip and corneal changes in the form of punctate epithelial erosions and filaments.

Diagnosis

Diagnosis of dry eye is confirmed when any two of the following three tests are positive :

1. *Tear film break-up (BUT)*. It is the interval between a complete blink and appearance of first randomly distributed dry spot on the cornea. It is noted after instilling a drop of fluorescein and examining in a cobalt-blue light of a slit-lamp. BUT is an indicator of adequacy of mucin component of tears. Its normal values range from 15-35 seconds. Values less than 10 seconds imply an unstable tear film.

2. *Schirmer-I test*. It measures total tear secretions. It is performed with the help of a 5 × 35 mm strip of Whatman-41 filter paper which is folded 5 mm from one end and kept in the lower fornix at the junction of lateral one-third and medial two-thirds. The patient is asked to look up and not to close the eyes. After 5 minutes wetting of the filter paper strip from the bent end is measured. Normal values of Schirmer-I test are more than 15 mm. Values of 5-10 mm are suggestive of moderate to mild keratoconjunctivitis sicca (KCS) and less than 5 mm of severe KCS.

3. *Rose Bengal staining* is a very useful test for detecting even mild care of dry eye. The devitalized dry conjunctival epithelial cells take up rose bengal stain.

Treatment
1. *Artificial tear drops* are instilled to treat dry eye. Artificial tears contain either methyl cellulose (0.7%) polyvinyl alcohol (1-1.7%).
2. *Occlusion of both punctae* help by preserving the existing tears in cases with severe dry eye.

THE WATERING EYE
The watering eye (overflow of tears) may occur either due to excessive secretion of tears (hyperlacrimation) or may result from obstruction to the outflow of normally secreted tears (epiphora).

Hyperlacrimation. It is usually the result of a reflex stimulation causing the gland to secrete more tears seen in almost all the inflammatory conditions of the eyeball and its adnexa.

Epiphora may occur due to obstruction at the level of puntum, canaliculi, lacrimal sac or nasolacrimal duct.

Clinical evaluation of a case of watering eye
1. *Examination with diffuse illumination using magnification* to rule out any cause of reflex hypersecretion and punctal causes of epiphora.
2. *Regurgitation test* is positive in patients with chronic dacryocystitis.
3. *Fluorescein dye disappearance test (FDDT)*. Normally one drop of fluorescein dye instilled into the conjunctival sac disappears within 2-3 minutes. A prolonged retention indicates obstruction to the flow of tears.
4. *Lacrimal syringing* (Fig. 14.2) is the most useful technique to test the potency of the lacrimal passages.

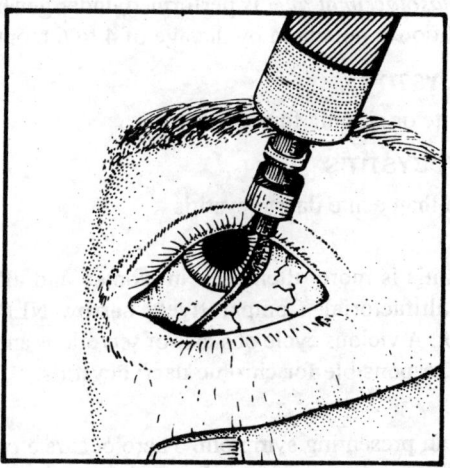

Fig. 14.2. Technique of lacrimal syringing.

5. *Dacryocystography.* In this technique the lacrimal passage are outlined with radio-opaque liquid, such as Lipiodal, so that exact site and nature of blockage can be examined radiographically.

DACRYOCYSTITIS

Inflammation of the lacrimal sac (dacryocystitis) is not an uncommon condition. It may occur in two forms congenital and adult dacryocystitis.

CONGENITAL DACRYOCYSTITIS

It is an inflammation of the lacrimal sac occurring in newborn infants, and is thus also known as *dacryocystitis neonatorum.*

Etiology

It follows non-drainage of tears because of congenital non-canalization of the lower end of nasolacrimal duct.

Clinical picture

It is characterized by watering from the eye, usually after first week of life. Soon it is followed by copious mucopurulent discharge from the eye with a positive regurgitation test.

Treatment

1. *Topical antibiotic drops* and pressure on the lacrimal sac area 3-4 times a day cures the condition in 80-90 percent of the infants.
2. *Lacrimal syringing* with saline and antibiotic solution should be performed if the condition is not cured by above treatment upto the age of 2 months. It helps to open the membranous occlusion by exerting hydraulic pressure.
3. *Probing of the nasolacrimal duct* is performed under general anaesthesia in case the condition is not cured by the age of 4 to 6 months.

ADULT DACRYOCYSTITS

It may occur in acute or chronic form.

CHRONIC DACRYOCYSTITIS

It is more common than acute dacryocystitis.

Etiology

Chronic dacryocystitis is more often seen in women and after middle age. The etiology is multifactorial. Comparatively narrow NLD is a common predispensing factor. A vicious cycle of stasis of secretions and mild infection of long duration is responsible for chronic dacryocystitis.

Clinical picture

Epiphora is the main presenting symptom. There occurs a *collection of pus or mucopus* in the lacrimal sac causing obstruction and regurgitation of the material. Chronic stagnation is followed by formation of *lacrimal mucocele* characterized by a visible swelling in the medial canthus (Fig. 14.3).

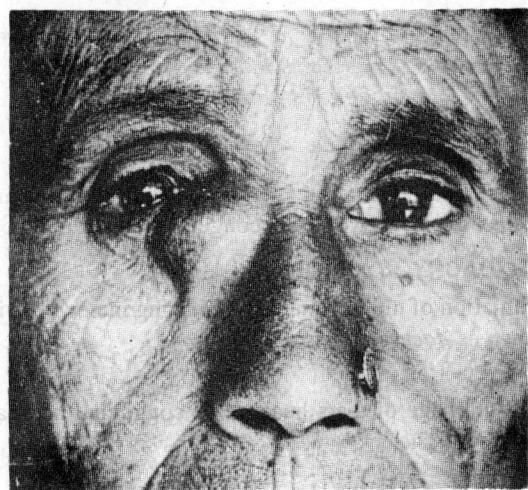

Fig. 14.3. Lacrimal mucocele.

Treatment

1. *Dacryocystorhinostomy (DCR)* operation in which the lacrimal sac is anastomosed to the nasal mucosa after removal of the portion of the intervening bone is usually required as an effective treatment.
2. *Dacryocystectomy* (DCT) ie. removal of lacrimal sac to prevent recurrent infection and complication is performed when DCR operation is contraindicated under following circumstances :
   - When the patient is too young (less than 4 years) or too old (more than 60 years).
   - When lacrimal sac is markedly shrunken and fibrosed .
   - When the sac is involved in tuberculosis, syphilis, leprosy or mycotic infection.
   - Gross nasal diseases like atrophic rhinitis.

Preoperative nursing care

1. *General preparation* for operation under general anaesthesia (see page 41).
2. *Local preparation* include packing of the nose with roll gauze soaked in solution of 4% xylocaine with adrenaline 1: 1000 to bring about constriction of blood vessels to reduce operative bleeding.

Postoperative nursing care

1. *General care* of a patient operated under general anaesthesia (see page 42).
2. *Observation* of the local dressed area for bleeding and soakage.
3. *Bandage is removed* after 24 - 48 hour and the wound is then left uncovered.
4. *Daily syringing* of the passages with normal saline begins an the third day after operation and continues until discharge from the hospital.

5. The patient should be advised not to blow his nose until healing has taken place.

ACUTE DACRYOCYSTITIS

It is an acute suppurative inflammation of the lacrimal sac.

Etiology

It may develop as an acute exacerbation of chronic dacryocystitis or as an acute peridacryocystitis due to direct involvement from the surrounding structures such as paranasal sinuses.

Clinical picture

It is characterized by a *painful swelling* in the region of lacrimal sac associated with *epiphora* and constitutional symptoms such as *fever* and *malaise*. Soon a *lacrimal abscess* is formed which points below and to the outer side of sac. If unattended the lacrimal abscess may discharge spontaneously leading to an *'external fistula'*.

Treatment

Systemic antibiotics and anti-inflammatory drugs along with local heat application is very useful. When abscess is formed, it needs to be drained.

Later, once the acute infection is treated, depending upon the condition of sac either DCT or DCR operation should be performed, otherwise, recurrence will occur.

15

Diseases of the Orbit

PROPTOSIS

It is defined as forward displacement of the eyeball beyond the orbital margins. Though the word *exophthalmos* (out eye) is synonymous with it; but somehow it has become customary to use the term exophthalmos for the outword displacement associated with thyroid disease.

Etiology

Any space-occupying lesion of the bony orbit will push the eyeball forward and cause proptosis. These lesions may be :

1. *Congenital* e.g., dermoid cyst.
2. *Traumatic* e.g., orbital haemorrhage
3. *Inflammatory* e.g. orbital cellulitis, cavernous sinus thrombosis, and pseudotumour.
4. *Tumour* of the orbit.
5. *Endocrinal disorder* e.g. thyroid eye disease.

Clinical features

1. Eyeball is pushed out. Proptosis may be unilateral or bilateral.
2. Lagophthalmos i.e. difficulty in closure of the eye if the proptosis is marked.

Treatment

Depends upon the cause of proptosis.

ORBITAL INFLAMMATIONS

ORBITAL CELLULITIS

It refers to purulent infection of the orbital cellular tissue. It is a serious condition.

Etiology

1. *Exogenous infection* may occur following peneterating wound of the orbit.

2. *Extension of infection* may occur from neighbouring structures such on paranasal sinuses. Ethmoiditis is the commonest cause of orbital cellulitis in children.

Clinical features

1. The patient appears to be acutely ill with fever, pain and prostration.
2. There is marked proptosis, conjunctival congestion and oedema of the lids (Fig. 15.1).
3. Abscess formation may either point to the skin of the eyelids or it may discharge through conjunctival fornix.

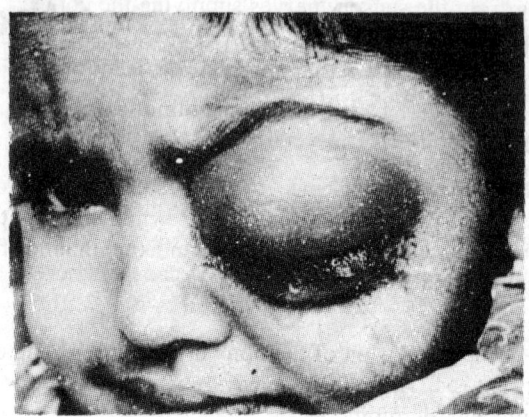

Fig. 15.1. Orbital cellulitis in a three-year-old female child.

Treatment

1. Intensive *antibiotics* to overcome infection.
2. Analgesics and anti-inflammatory drugs.
3. Surgical incision and drainage may be required when the abscess is formed.

Nursing care

1. Nursing care of an acutely ill patient is required with every four hour record of temperature, pulse and respiration.
2. Local heat application may relieve some discomfort.
3. The patient should be nursed in bed in whatever position he finds to be most comfortable.
4. He must be encouraged to drink plenty of fluids and though a light diet may be given during the first few days of acute illness the patient may have no appetite.

CAVERNOUS SINUS THROMBOSIS

Septic thrombosis of the cavernous sinus is a disastrous sequel resulting from spread of sepsis travelling along its tributaries.

Etiology

Cavernous sinus thrombosis can occur as a complication of orbital cellulitis or as a result of spread of infection from the other surrounding structures in the area of head and neck.

Clinical picture

1. *General features.* Patient is critically ill owing high grade fever with rigors, vomiting and headache.
2. *Ocular features.* There occurs *proptosis* conjunctival congestion and chemosis, palsy of ocular motor nerves and insensitivity of the cornea resulting from the sensory nerves supplying the cornea.

Treatment

The outcome can prove fatal unless intensive treatment is undertaken.

1. *Antibiotics.* Modern broad spectrum antibiotics injected intravenously are required to treat the infection.
2. *Analgesics and anti-inflammatory* drugs control pain and fever.
3. Role of *anticoagulants* is controversial.

Nursing care

1. General nursing care of a critically ill patient is required. Nursing care aims at making the patient as comfortable as is possible, both physically and mentally.
2. Patient needs complete nursing care in the bed including the recording of temperature, pulse and respiration every four hourly.
3. Pressure area should be treated four hourly and attention paid to oral toilet.
4. A daily bed bath should be given.

GRAVES' OPHTHALMOPATHY

Graves' ophthalmopathy or the ocular Graves' disease refers to typical ocular changes which include lid retraction, lid lag and proptosis (Fig. 15.2).

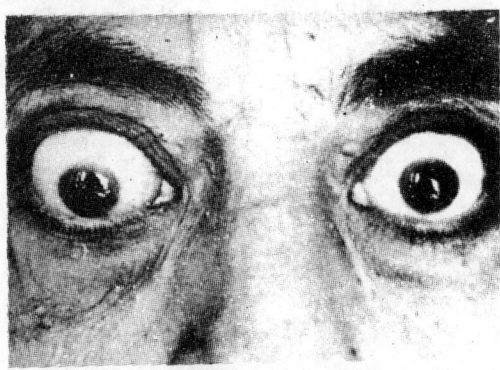

Fig. 15.2. A patient with Graves' ophthalmopathy having bilateral exophthalmos and lid retraction.

Etiology

It may be a part of Graves' disease (Hyperthyroidism) or may be associated with hypothyroidism or even euthyroidism. It is now suggested that Graves' ophthalmopathy has an autoimmune etiology.

Clinical features

1. *Thyrotoxic exophthalmos.* In this form a mild exophthalmos is associated with lid lag, lid retraction and all signs of thyrotoxicosis which include, tachycardia, muscular tremors and raised basal metabolism.

2. *Thyrotropic exophthalmos.* In this clinical variety an extreme exophthalmos and external ophthalmoplegia (due to infiltrative thyroid ophthalmopathy) are associated with euthyroidism or hypothyroidism. The condition usually affects middle-aged persons and runs a self-limiting course characterized by remissions and relapses.

Management

1. *Thyrotoxicosis* when associated should be treated.
2. *Artificial tear drops* are useful for symptoms of ocular surface drying.
3. *Systemic steroids* may be indicated in patients with rapidly progressive chemosis and proptosis.
4. *Radiotherapy* may be required where steroids are contraindicated.
5. *Lateral tarsorrhaphy* should be performed in patients with exposure keratitis.
6. *Surgical decompression* is indicated in patients with imminent danger of permanent visual loss.

ORBITAL TUMOURS

Orbital tumours are not very common. These may be primary, secondary and metastatic tumours. Primary tumour may be benign or malignant and may arise from the walls or contents of the orbit. They usually present with proptosis and are managed depending upon the type and extent of the growth.

16

Ocular Injuries

MECHANICAL INJURIES

In this era of high speed traffic and industrialization, the incidence of injuries is increasing in general. Like any other part of the body eyes are also not exempt from these injuries. A staff nurse not only has to assist the ophthalmologists in the management but sometimes may be the first person to attend the emergency. So she needs to be well versed with the first aid care which is often virtually important and may prevent blindness. Mechanical injuries can be grouped as under :

1. Retained extraocular foreign bodies
2. Blunt trauma (Contusional injury)
3. Penetrating and perforating injuries
4. Penetrating injuries with retained intraocular foreign bodies.

EXTRAOCULAR FOREIGN BODIES

Conjunctival and corneal foreign bodies are the commonest of all eye injuries. Because of the great discomfort, watering and even pain produced by the foreign bodies, patients usually report in the emergency department. Particles lying upon the conjunctiva are not of serious significance and may safely be cared for by the first-aider which may be a staff nurse. However, foreign bodies on the cornea must be removed by a physician. A sterile local anaesthetic is instilled into the eye and the foreign body is removed with a swab stick, hypodermic needle or special foreign body spud. After the foreign body is removed, an antibiotic ointment is instilled and patching is done for 24 hours. Antibiotic eye drops are instilled 3-4 times a day for a week. Untreated corneal infection is serious.

BLUNT TRAUMA

Blunt trauma to the eyes may occur following a direct blow to the eye by fist, ball or blunt object like sticks. It may also occur in accidents.

Blunt trauma causes contusional injuries which may vary in severity from a simple corneal abrasion to an extensive rupture of globe which need to be managed as follows :

1. *Abrasions of the cornea* may be treated with an antibiotic ointment prophylactically and an eye bandage applied with firm gentle pressure.

2. *Contusion of the eyeball* i.e. closed globe trauma with injury to intraocular structures with intraocular haemorrhage need a careful evaluation and management.
   - Complete bed rest for 6-7 days is required
   - Intraocular pressure, when raised must be lowered by use of topical 0.5% timolol eye drops, oral aetazolamide or even intravenous mannitol.
   - *Topical and systemic steroids* are useful in treating traumatic inflammation.
   - *Cycloplegics* like homatropine are also useful for the management of uveitis.

3. *Rupture of the globe* needs meticulous repair. A badly mutilated eyeball should be enucleated.

PENETRATING AND PERFORATING INJURIES

Penetrating injury refers to a single full thickness laceration of the eyewall caused by a sharp object. While perforating injury refers to two full thickness wounds (one entry and one exit) of the eyewall caused by a sharp object or missile.

Such injuries can cause severe damage to the eye and should be treated as serious emergencies. In addition to mechanical lacerating effects of trauma, introduction of infection, post traumatic iridocyclitis and sympathetic ophthalmitis are serious potential complications of peneterating injuries.

Treatment

A meticulous repair of the wound with abscission of the prolapsed uveal tissue (if any) should be carried out immediately. Intensive antibiotic therapy and topical steroids and cycloplegics should be given after the repair. A severely wounded eye should be enucleated.

INTRAOCULAR FOREIGN BODIES

In addition to the above mentioned serious effects of penetrating injuries, retained intraocular foreignbody (RIOFB) carries the risk of reaction caused by the foreign body. The specific reaction (degenerative changes in the eye tissue) caused by a retained iron foreign body is known as *'siderosis bulbi'* and that caused by a copper foreign body is *chalcosis*. Therefore, a case with retained IOFB requires immediate evaluation by an ophthalmologist. The efforts should be made to remove the IOFB as early as possible.

Important points in Nursing care of a patient with ocular injuries

1. Always wash your hands thoroughly before approaching the eye.

2. Eyes with surface foreign bodies should not be rubbed.
3. Avoid applying pressure on the eye and also do not allow the patient to do so.
4. Penetrating injuries may be covered with a plastic or metal eyeshield to protect the eye until the patient is seen by the doctor.
5. Remember to use sterile medications and sterile technique whenever a penetrating injury has occurred.
6. Tetanus prophylaxis should be given routinely to all patients with penetrating injuries.
7. Advise the patient not to eat or drink until ophthalmologist gives any instructions, because surgical repairs of peneterating injuries are usually performed under general anaesthesia.

NON-MECHNICAL INJUIRES

CHEMICAL INJURIES

Chemical injuires are by no means uncommon.

Causes

These usually occur due to external contact with chemicals under following circumstances :
1. *Domestic accidents,* e.g. with ammonia, solvents, detergents and cosmetics.
2. *Agricultural accidents,* e.g. due to fertilizers, insecticides, toxins of vegetable and animal origin.
3. *Chemical laboratory accidents,* with acids and alkalies.
4. *Deliberate chemical attacks,* especially with acids to disfigure the face.
5. *Chemical warfare* injuries.
6. *Self-inflicted chemical* injuries are seen in malingerers and psychopaths.

Clinical features

In general alkali burns are more damaging than the acid burns. Extent of damage depends upon the concentration of chemical. *Immediate lesions* are:
1. *Conjunctiva* shows marked oedema congestion and wide spread necrosis.
2. *Cornea* develops widespread sloughing of the epithelium, oedema and opalescence.
3. *Iris and ciliary body* and inflammed in severe alkali burns.
   After a few days cornea may be vascularized, symblepharon and corneal ulceration may occur.

Treatment

1. Regardless of the type of chemical injury the emergency treatment is always immediate and prolonged washing of the eye with plain water.

2. Next all particles of foreign matter should be removed under topical anaesthesia.
3. Topical antibiotics and corticosteroids are instilled to prevent infection and scarring.
4. Atropine drops / ointment should be instilled to take care of the iridocyclitis.
5. Symblepharon formation should be prevented by frequently sweeping a glass rod in the fornices.

17

Systemic Ophthalmology

Ocular involvement in systemic disorders is quite frequent. It is imperative for the nurses to be well conversant with these, since they may come across such a situation while working in different wards. Therefore, ocular lesions of the common systemic disorders are enumerated and a few important ones are described here.

OCULAR MANIFESTATIONS OF NUTRITIONAL DEFICIENCES

1. *Deficiency of vitamin A*. Ocular manifestations of vitamin A deficiency are referred to as xerophthalmia.
2. *Deficiency of vitamin B₁ (thiamine)*. It can cause corneal anaesthesia, conjunctival and corneal dystrophy and acute retrobulbar neuritis.
3. *Deficiency of vitamin B₂ (riboflavin)*. It can produce photophobia and burning sensation in the eyes due to conjunctival irritation and vascularisation of the cornea.
4. *Deficiency of vitamin C*. It may be associated with haemorrhages in the conjunctiva, lids, anterior chamber, retina and orbit. It also delays wound healing.
5. *Deficiency of vitamin D*. It may be associated with zonular cataract, papilloedema and increased lacrimation.

XEROPHTHALMIA

It is a term now reserved (by a joint WHO and USAID Committee, in 1976) to cover all the ocular manifestations of vitamin A deficiency.

Etiology

It occurs either due to *dietary deficiency* of vitamin A or its *defective absorption* from the gut. It has long been recognised that vitamin A deficiency does not occur as an isolated problem but is almost invariably accompanied by protein-energy malnutrition (PEM) and infections.

Clinical features *(WHO classification,1982)*

The new xerophthalmia classification (modification of original 1976 classification) is as follows:

XN	:	Night blindness
X1A	:	Conjunctival xerosis
X1B	:	Bitot's spots (Pl. III. 6)
X2	:	Corneal xerosis
X3A	:	Corneal ulceration/keratomalacia affecting less than one-third corneal surface
X3B	:	Corneal ulceration/keratomalacia affecting more than one-third corneal surface.
XS	:	Corneal scar due to xerophthalmia
XF	:	Xerophthalmic fundus.

Treatment

Vitamin A therapy.

1. *All patients above the age of 1 year* (except women of reproductive age): 200,000 IU of vitamin A orally or 100,000 IU by intramuscular injection should be given immediately on diagnosis and repeated the following day and 4 weeks later.
2. *Children under the age of 1 year and children of any age who weigh less than 8 kg* should be treated with half the doses for patients of more than 1 year of age.
3. *Women of reproductive age, pregnant or not:* (a) *Those having night blindness* (XN), conjunctival xerosis (X1A) and Bitot's spots (X1B) should be treated with a daily dose of 10,000 IU of vitamin A orally (1 sugar coated tablet) for 2 weeks. (b) *For corneal xerophthalmia,* administration of full dosage schedule (described for patients above 1 year of age) is recommended.

Prophylaxis against xerophthalmia

WHO recommended, universal distribution schedule of vitamin A for prevention is as follows (also see page 433-434) :

i. Infants 6-12 months old and any older children who weigh less than 8 kg.	100,000 IU orally every 3-6 months.
ii. Children over 1 year and under 6 years of age	200,000 IU orally every 6 months.

| iii. Lactating | 20,000 IU orally once at mothers delivery or during the next 2 months. This will raise the concentration of vitamin A in the breast milk and therefore, help to protect the breastfed infant. |
| iv. Infants less than 6 months old, not being breast-fed. | 50,000 IU orally should be given before they attain the age of 6 months. |

OCULAR MANIFESTATIONS OF SYSTEMIC INFECTIONS

A. Viral infections

1. *Measles.* Ocular lesions are: catarrhal conjunctivitis, Koplik's spots on conjunctiva, corneal ulceration, optic neuritis and retinitis.

2. *Mumps.* Ocular involvement may occur as conjunctivitis, keratitis, acute dacryoadenitis and uveitis.

3. *Rubella.* Ocular lesions seen in rubella (German measles) are congenital microphthalmos, cataract, glaucoma, chorioretinitis and optic atrophy.

4. *Whooping cough.* There may occur subconjunctival haemorrhages and rarely orbital haemorrhage leading to proptosis.

5. *Ocular involvement in AIDS.* AIDS (Acquired Immune Deficiency Syndrome) is caused by Human immunodeficiency virus (HIV) which is an RNA retrovirus.

Ocular lesions of AIDS may be classified as follows:

1. *Retinal microvasculopathy.* It develops from vaso-occlusive process which may be either due to direct toxic effects of virus on the vascular endothelium or immune complex deposits in the precapillary arterioles.

2. *Usual ocular infections.* These are also seen in healthy people, but occur with greater frequency and produce more severe infections in patients with AIDS. These include herpes zoster ophthalmicus, herpes simplex infections, toxoplasmosis (chorioretinitis), ocular tuberculosis, syphilis and fungal corneal ulcers.

3. *Opportunistic infections of the eye.* These are caused by microorganisms which do not affect normal patients. They can infect someone whose cellular immunity is suppressed by HIV infection or by other causes such as leukaemia. These include: cytomegalovirus (CMV) retinitis, candida endophthalmitis, cryptococcal infections and pneumocystis carinii, choroiditis.

4. *Unusual neoplasms* include. Kaposi's sarcoma of eyelids or conjunctiva and Burkitt's lymphoma of the orbit.

5. *Neuro-ophthalmic lesions.* These include isolated or multiple cranial nerve palsies.

B. Bacterial Infections

1. *Septicaemia.* Ocular involvement may occur in the form of metastatic retinitis, uveitis or endophthalmitis.

2. *Diphtheria.* There may occur: membranous conjunctivitis, corneal ulceration, paralysis of accommodation and paralysis of extraocular muscles.

3. *Brucellosis.* It may involve the eye in the form of iritis, choroiditis and optic neuritis.

4. *Gonococcal ocular lesions* are: ophthalmia neonatorum, acute purulent conjunctivitis in adults and corneal ulceration.

5. *Meningococcal infection* may be associated with: metastatic conjunctivitis, corneal ulceration, paresis of extraocular muscles, optic neuritis and metastatic endophthalmitis or panophthalmitis.

6. *Typhoid fever.* It may be complicated by optic neuritis and corneal ulceration due to lagophthalmos.

7. *Tuberculosis.* Ocular lesions seen are granulomatous conjunctivitis, phlyctenular keratoconjunctivitis, interstitial keratitis, nongranulomatous and granulomatous uveitis, Eales' disease, optic atrophy (following chiasmal arachnoiditis secondary to meningitis), and papilloedema (due to raised intracranial pressure following intracranial tuberculoma).

8. *Syphilitic lesions* (acquired) seen in *primary stage* are conjunctivitis and chancre of conjunctiva. In *secondary stage* there may occur iridocyclitis. *Tertiary stage* lesions include chorioretinitis and gummata in the orbit. *Neurosyphilis* is associated with optic atrophy and pupillary abnormalities. Ocular lesions of *congenital syphilis* are: interstitial keratitis, iridocyclitis and chorioretinitis.

9. *Leprosy.* Ocular lesions of leprosy include cutaneous nodules on the eyelids, madarosis, interstitial keratitis, exposure keratitis, granulomatous uveitis and dacryocystitis.

C. Parasitic infections

1. *Toxoplasmosis* is known to produce necrotising chorioretinitis.

2. *Taenia echinococcus* infestation may manifest as hydatid cyst of the orbit, vitreous and retina.

3. *Taenia solium* infestation. Cysticercus cysts are known to involve conjunctiva, vitreous, retina, orbit and extra-ocular muscles.

4. *Toxocara* infestation may be associated with endophthalmitis.

D. Fungal infections

Systemic fungal infections may be associated with corneal ulceration and endophthalmitis.

OCULAR MANIFESTATIONS OF COMMON METABOLIC DISORDERS

Gout

Ocular lesions of gout include: episcleritis, scleritis and uveitis.

Diabetes mellitus

Ocular involvement in diabetes is very common. Structure-wise ocular lesions are as follows:

1. *Lids*: Xanthelasma and recurrent stye or internal hordeolum
2. *Conjunctiva*: Telangiectasia, sludging of the blood in conjunctival vessels and subconjunctival haemorrhage
3. *Cornea*: Pigment dispersal at back of cornea, decreased corneal sensations (due to trigeminal neuropathy), punctate kerotapathy, Descemet's folds, higher incidence of infective corneal ulcers and delayed epithelial healing due to abnormality in epithelial basement membrane
4. *Iris*: Rubeosis iridis (neovascularization)
5. *Lens*: Snow-flake cataract in patients with IDDM, posterior subcapsular cataract, early onset and maturation of senile cataract
6. *Vitreous*: Vitreous haemorrhage and fibro- vascular proliferation secondary to diabetic retinopathy
7. *Retina:* Diabetic retinopathy and lipaemia retinalis
8. *Intraocular pressure*: Increased incidence of POAG, neovascular glaucoma and hypotony in diabetic ketoacidosis (due to increased plasma bicarbonate levels)
9. *Optic nerve* : Optic neuritis
10. *Extraocular muscles*: Ophthalmoplegia due to diabetic neuropathy
11. *Changes in refraction*: Hypermetropic shift in hypoglycemia, myopic shift in hyperglycemia and decreased accommodation

Galactosemia

It is usually associated with congenital cataract.

Homocystinuria

It is associated with bilateral subluxation of lens.

OCULAR MANIFESTATIONS OF COMMON DISORDERS OF SKIN AND MUCOUS MEMBRANES

1. *Atopic dermatitis.* It may be associated with conjunctivitis, keratoconus and cataract.
2. *Rosacea.* Its ocular lesions include blepharitis, conjunctivitis, keratitis and rosacea pannus.

3. *Dermatitis herpetiformis.* Its ocular complications include recurrent bullae, ulceration and cicatrization.

4. *Epidermolysis bullosa.* Ocular complications, when they occur, take the form of cicatrizing conjunctivitis and keratitis.

OCULAR MANIFESTATIONS OF DISEASES OF CENTRAL NERVOUS SYSTEM

Ocular involvement in diseases of the central nervous system is not infrequent and may occur in almost all the disorders which include intracranial infection, aneurysms harmorrhage, tumours and demyelinating disorders.

Common ocular manifestations are :

– Papilloedema
– Optic neuritis
– Palsy of 3rd, 4th and 6th cranial nerves.
– Pupillary abnormalities.

18

Community Ophthalmology

Community ophthalmology aims at promoting ocular health and preventing blindness at the community level with an active, recognized and crucial role of community participation. A staff nurse has to play an important role in promoting the concept of community ophthalmology. So she needs to be familiar with the community eye health problems, working of the 'National Programme for Control of Blindness' and the care and rehabilitation of a blind person.

BLINDNESS AND ITS CAUSES

DEFINITION OF BLINDNESS

WHO has defined blindness as, "visual acuity of less than 3/60 (Snellens) or its equivalent in the better eye." While the term *'visual impairment'* is used when the maximum vision in the better eye is 6/18 (Snellens).

Preventable blindness is that which can be easily prevented by attacking the causative factor at an appropriate time. For example corneal blindness due to vitamin A deficiency can be prevented by timely use of vitamin - A while in *curable blindness* vision can be restored by timely intervention. For example cataract blindness can be cured by surgical treatment.

MAGNITUDE OF BLINDNESS

Global blindness. Presently an estimated 180 million people worldwide are visually disabled of whom nearly 45 million are blind, four out of five of them living in developing nations.

Blindness in India. Presently in India there are about 12 million blind people, which comes to more than one-fourth of the total blinds in the world. According to WHO-NPCB survey (1986-89) the prevalence of blindness in India is 1.49%.

CAUSES OF BLINDNESS IN INDIA

The main causes of blindness in India, estimated by WHO-NPCB survey (1986-89) are as below :

Cataract	80.10%
Refractive errors	7.35 %
Aphakic blindness	4.67 %
Glaucoma	1.70%
Corneal opacity	1.52%
Trachoma	0.39%
Other	4.25%

NATIONAL PROGRAMME FOR CONTROL OF BLINDNESS

Objectives

The 'National Programme for Control of Blindness' (NPCB) was formulated and launched as a 100% centrally sponsored scheme in 1976 with following objectives :

1. To provide comprehensive eye care facilities for primary, secondary and tertiary levels of eye health care.
2. To reduce the prevalence of blindness.

Plan of action and activities

1. *Extension of eye care services* through eye camps in the remote areas.
2. *Establishment of permanent infrastructure* for primary eye care in primary health centres, for secondary eye care at district and tehsil hospitals and for tertiary eye care in Medical Colleges and Regional Institutes of Ophthalmology.
3. *Intensification of eye health education* through mass communication media, school teachers, social workers and community leaders.
4. *Specific programme* under NPCB to cover important area are :
   - Trachoma control programme
   - School eye health services
   - Vitamin A prophylaxis programme
   - Occupational eye-health services
   - World Bank assisted cataract blindness control project

Programme organization

1. *Central level* control and planning is done at the office of 'Director General Health Services, Govt of India'.
2. *State level* implementation of the NPCB is done through state programme cell of the respective state governments.
3. *District level.* To organize and implement various activitis of NPCB at district level, 'District Blindness Control Societies' (DBCS) are being established.

REHABILITATION OF THE BLIND

It is as important as the prevention and control of blindness; spiritually speaking even more. A blind person needs the following types of rehabilitation.

1. *Medical rehabilitation.* By low vision aids (LVA) many visually handicapped can have a useful vision.

2. *Training and psychosocial rehabilitation.* It is the most important aspect. First of all each blind should be assured and made to feel that they are equally useful and not inferior to the sighted persons. Their training should include:
   i. Mobility training with the help of a stick.
   ii. Training in daily living skills, such as bathing washing, putting on clothes, shaving, cooking and other household work.

3. *Educational rehabilitation.* It includes education avenues in Blind schools with the facility of Braille system of education.

4. *Vocational rehabilitation.* It will help them to earn their livelihood and live as useful citizens. Blinds can be trained in making handicrafts, canning, book binding, candle and chalk making, cottage industries and as telephone operators.

To conclude, it should never be forgotten that, one of the basic human rights is the right to see. The strategicians MUST ensure that :
- No citizen goes blind needlessly due to preventable causes.
- All avenues are exhausted to restore the best possible vision to curable blinds.
- Blinds not amenable to curable measures receive comprehensive rehabilitation.

NURSE AS A COMMUNITY EYE HEALTH WORKER

A nurse has to play an important role in promoting the concept of community and preventive ophthalmology. Since eye health education forms a vital component of measures for the prevention and cure of avoidable blindness, a nurse should be fully prepared to impart eye health education to the patients and their attendents. Eye health education should be given with particular refrence to :

1. *Prevention of communicable eye diseases* like trachoma and conjunctivitis. People should be taught about the ways these diseases spread and the meaures to prevent them (see page.90).A proper personal hygiene and improved sanitation can prevent from many communicable diseases.

2. *Prevention of nutritional blindness.* Nutritional blindness can be reduced, if not eliminated, if the people are educated about the value

of vitamin A and the food articles which provide this vitamin. People should be taught to include green leaf vegetables, yellow colour vegetables likes sitaphal, and fruits like mango, papaya etc. in diet. Leaves of drumstick also provide good amount of vitamin A (also see page 195).

3. *Occupational hazards to the eyesight and their prevention.* Farmers and field workers and those engaged in stone cutting and welding industries should be advised to wear protective glasses while at work.

4. *For early detection of visual defects,* parents should be advised to get the eyes of their children checked at school entry. The early detection of visual defects is very important to prevent permanent visual loss.

5. *Visual hygiene.* School children should be taught about the visual hygiene with particular refrence to adequate lighting and proper posture during reading.

6. *Information about glaucoma and other blinding diseases* should be given to the people for their timely intervention.

7. *Advise to beware of eye quacks and harmful eye medicines* especially various types of poor quality surmas should be given to the people.

8. *Information about eye care health services.* People should be made aware of the eye care health services available to them. In villages, many patients with cataract even hesitate to go for surgery for fear of operation. Health education should aim at removing such fears and encourage people to come forward for operations.

9. *Education for voluntary eye donations.* People should be taught and made aware about voluntary eye donations.

Index